T0291004

An Interprofessional Approach to
Veterinary Nutrition

An Interprofessional Approach to Veterinary Nutrition

Rachel H. Lumbis and Tierney Kinnison

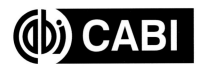

CABI is a trading name of CAB International

CABI	CABI
Nosworthy Way	200 Portland Street
Wallingford	Boston
Oxfordshire OX10 8DE	MA 02114
UK	USA
Tel: +44 (0)1491 832111	Tel: +1 (617)682-9015
E-mail: info@cabi.org	E-mail: cabi-nao@cabi.org
Website: www.cabi.org	

The views expressed in this publication are those of the author(s) and do not necessarily represent those of, and should not be attributed to, CAB International (CABI). Any images, figures and tables not otherwise attributed are the author(s)' own. References to internet websites (URLs) were accurate at the time of writing.

CAB International and, where different, the copyright owner shall not be liable for technical or other errors or omissions contained herein. The information is supplied without obligation and on the understanding that any person who acts upon it, or otherwise changes their position in reliance thereon, does so entirely at their own risk. Information supplied is neither intended nor implied to be a substitute for professional advice. The reader/user accepts all risks and responsibility for losses, damages, costs and other consequences resulting directly or indirectly from using this information.

CABI's Terms and Conditions, including its full disclaimer, may be found at https://www.cabi.org/terms-and-conditions/.

A catalogue record for this book is available from the British Library, London, UK.

ISBN-13: 9781800621084 (paperback)
       9781800621091 (ePDF)
       9781800621107 (ePub)

DOI: 10.1079/9781800621107.0000

Commissioning Editor: Alexandra Lainsbury
Editorial Assistant: Lauren Davies
Production Editor: James Bishop

Typeset by Straive, Pondicherry, India
Printed and bound in the USA by Integrated Books International, Dulles, Virginia

The time, commitment and vision needed to complete this project would not have been possible without the support, guidance and inspiration from our families (including pets), friends, colleagues, mentors and patients.

Contents

Foreword by Dr Cecilia Villaverde Haro

A good nutritional and feeding management of companion animals is very important to maintain their health and longevity; both as part of preventative medicine and to manage disease conditions, acute and chronic. As a veterinary nutrition specialist, I have seen that caretakers are more aware of the importance of good nutrition than ever and want the right feeding plan for their pet. However, this can be very challenging, since there are so many options available. The veterinary healthcare team (VHCT) is, therefore, an invaluable resource in this regard. However, performing a nutritional assessment and providing lifelong feeding recommendations is complex and not always done or, if done, the advice is not always followed by the caretakers. It is important to know the reasons why, and then implement strategies to provide adequate nutritional advice to all the patients.

This book provides practical solutions to these challenges centred on the importance of interprofessional practice and teamwork. I especially appreciate that one of the overarching themes here is communication: both among the different professionals involved in vet care and with the pet caretakers. While effective communication is always important, its role in veterinary nutrition care cannot be overstated. Nutrition is a difficult and emotional topic to discuss, including weight management, and there are many prevalent myths and misinformation about best nutrition for pets. Having more tools for the whole team to communicate among themselves, the clients, and any other external individuals can only help improve the nutritional management and, therefore, overall health, of our patients.

The authors of this book have the experience and credentials to provide excellent advice to enable the VHCT to implement nutrition care for their patients. I am very excited about this book becoming a valuable resource for all of us.

Dr Cecilia Villaverde Haro, BVSc, PhD, Diplomate (Nutrition) of the ACVIM (Board-Certified Veterinary Nutritionist), Diplomate ECVCN (EBVS European Specialist in Veterinary and Comparative Nutrition)

2 January 2023

Foreword by Professor Stephen May

If the 20th century is characterised (justifiably) as the age of the individual expert, or group of experts in a single domain, the 21st century must be seen as the age in which interdisciplinary expert teams should dominate and thrive. News media bombard us daily with yet more complex problems, searching solutions that elude individual experts. Whether we are dealing with the health problems of animals and people that involve more than one organ system, or global economic/social/health/political issues, individual specialists are often too narrow in their expertise to deal with these levels of complexity.

However, creation of an interdisciplinary expert team is not as simple as putting together groups of individual subject specialists, from different relevant disciplines, as the subsequent chapters in this book reveal. Each member of an interdisciplinary team needs knowledge of the areas of expertise of the other members and the synergies that may be created by members working well together. This knowledge has been described as 'interactional expertise' (Collins *et al.*, 2007); such an expert does not have the practical skills to work in an area, but they understand how the specialist in the other discipline generates new knowledge. Left to their own devices, individual subject experts are prone to 'cognitive entrenchment' (Dane, 2010), which means that they become inflexible and are blinded to methods and knowledge outside their domain. Such specialists can be a liability in teams involved in complex problem-solving. In contrast, experts with interactional expertise are able to engage in 'team cognition' (Salas *et al.*, 2007), mobilising their own expertise, and drawing on that of others, to contribute to combined decisions on ways to move forward. Further, research involving political forecasting has demonstrated that those with appropriate cognitive mindsets, including 'fluid intelligence', that open them to new possibilities, improve as 'superforecasters' if they repeatedly work in likeminded teams (Mellers *et al.*, 2015).

The modern veterinary (like the modern medical) team is a good example of how interdisciplinary working can lead to better management solutions for complex problems. This is well illustrated by the central role of nutrition to health, and the increasingly well recognised improvements in prognoses, for both acute and chronic conditions, if all healthcare team members collaborate in ensuring individual nutritional component needs, as well as overall nutritional needs, are met. I am sure volumes such as this represent a new beginning in the literature aimed at advancing veterinary care, and the authors are to be congratulated in bringing their research on interdisciplinary working to the attention of the broader veterinary audience.

Professor Stephen May MA VetMB PhD DVR DEO FRCVS DipECVS FHEA
Senior Vice-Principal Royal Veterinary College, University of London
RCVS Council Member

21 December 2022

References

Collins, H., Evans, R. and Gorman, M. (2007) Trading zones and interactional expertise. *Studies In History and Philosophy of Science Part A*, 38(4), 657–666.

Dane, E. (2010) Reconsidering the trade-off between expertise and flexibility: A cognitive entrenchment perspective. *Academy of Management Review*, 35(4), 579–603.

Mellers, B., Stone, E., Murray, T., Minster, A., Rohrbaugh, N., Bishop, M., Chen, E., Baker, J., Hou, Y., Horowitz, M., Ungar, L. and Tetlock, P. (2015) Identifying and cultivating superforecasters as a method of improving probabilistic predictions. *Perspectives on Psychological Science*, 10(3), 267–281.

Salas, E., Rosen, M.A., Burke, C.S., Nicholson, D. and Howse, W.R. (2007) Markers for enhancing team cognition in complex environments: the power of team performance diagnosis. *Aviation, Space, and Environmental Medicine*, 78(5 Suppl.), B77–85.

Preface

Awareness and appreciation of the importance of effective interprofessional practice and nutritional assessment is lacking in veterinary practice and the authors are keen to help address this. In veterinary practice, the interface between veterinarians, veterinary nurses, technicians, support staff and paraprofessional team members is crucial. It influences patient care and outcomes, the incidence of medical errors, client satisfaction, the success of the veterinary practice and the generation of revenue. Ensuring a coherent approach to the maintenance of the health and wellbeing of animals committed to veterinary care should be of paramount importance and involve the delegation of work according to relevant skills, competence and expertise. This requires an underlying basis of understanding, trust and respect between interprofessional members of the team.

Nutrition is one of the most important considerations in the maintenance of health and plays a critical role in the management of diseases, patient recovery and hospital outcome; a reflection of its acknowledgment as the fifth vital assessment in the standard patient examination after temperature, pulse, respiration and pain. Maintaining the health of pets through the provision of correct nutrition is an essential component of responsible pet ownership and one that caretakers are becoming increasingly aware of as a key factor in optimising pet health and wellbeing. Yet considerable confusion and misinformation exists regarding nutritional facts and dietary choice, with many caretakers finding this the most difficult aspect of pet ownership. Consequently, incorrect dietary decision-making by pet caretakers has the potential to cause harm to animals.

The veterinary healthcare team have a central role as the expert source of nutritional information, with each member capable of playing an important part in providing appropriate nutritional support and recommendations. The authors are cognisant of the acknowledged challenges to the provision of optimal nutritional care and advice in veterinary practice. Yet effective interprofessional communication and collaboration is a key factor in the successful implementation of nutritional assessment, delivery of nutritional support and in maximising the effectiveness of pet food recommendations. It leads to a positive team environment founded on respect, trust and mutual support and can help to overcome such challenges, facilitating the consistent implementation and record of nutritional assessment, planning and recommendations for every veterinary patient.

The overall aim of this book is to support veterinary healthcare teams in implementing optimal interprofessional and evidence-based approaches to nutritional care and support for their individual situations. Further objectives are to:

- discuss the underpinning theoretical and practical knowledge that veterinary professionals need to cultivate interprofessional practice
- explore the factors that influence the collaborative potential of the veterinary healthcare team
- demonstrate how robust interprofessional practice and teamwork can help to overcome challenges in providing nutritional care and advice
- highlight the veterinary healthcare team as the primary resource for sound nutritional advice.

There is an extensive range of publications dedicated to the topic of veterinary nutrition for healthy and diseased animals and designed for the veterinary healthcare team, paraprofessionals and pet caretakers. It is beyond the scope of this book to duplicate this information within, but readers are signposted throughout to recommended further reading and nutrition-related resources.

It is our sincere hope that this book will prove an invaluable resource to all members of the veterinary healthcare team and support staff, as well as to students, educators, industry representatives and paraprofessionals, and that a proactive attitude to nutrition will be adopted.

Acknowledgements

Rachel H. Lumbis and Tierney Kinnison

With many thanks to Dr Cecilia Villaverde Haro and Professor Stephen May for taking the considerable time and effort necessary to review the manuscript. We sincerely appreciate their constructive and insightful comments and suggestions which have helped to enhance the quality of the book.

Thanks also to Cecilia, Emma Davies, Emma Rees, Matthew Rendle and Terri Bussi, for sharing their thoughts and inspiration for the patient scenarios, and to all the interprofessional team members and colleagues who have contributed to the research which is presented in this book. Without your input, we would not be able to learn about veterinary teamworking and help the veterinary teams of today and tomorrow.

We are also extremely thankful to the editorial team at CABI for their initial invitation to write this book and for their patience, guidance and encouragement during the publishing process. We are especially grateful to Alex Lainsbury, Ali Thompson, Alison Smith and Lauren Davies of CABI and copy editor Jonathan Ingoldby, for their assistance in progressing this book from initial idea through to publication and beyond.

Rachel H. Lumbis

Thank you to my family and friends for their unconditional love, support and encouragement, in particular C.E.L and P.M.L., whose interest in this, as in all my endeavours, has never been less than my own and to whom I owe so much; A.J.S for optimising *my* dietary intake; E.P.S for being the light in my life.

Many thanks also to Professor Daniel Chan, Dr Isuru Gajanayake and the many colleagues I've worked with on the WSAVA Global Nutrition Committee and the European Veterinary Nutrition Educators Group who have shared their passion for, and knowledge of, veterinary nutrition with me.

Tierney Kinnison

Thank you to all my wonderful family and friends who have supported me throughout my education and work, as well as my exceptional current and past RVC colleagues who have taught me so much and who are helping to drive forwards interprofessional education in veterinary schools.

Introduction

1

Tierney Kinnison

Abstract
This short introduction outlines the aims of this book and provides a definition of 'interprofessional'. A brief explanation of why it is important to consider interprofessional practice is included alongside clarification of the sources from which the evidence base for this book is derived.

We are delighted that you are reading this book on an interprofessional approach to nutrition. The overall aim of this book is to provide evidence-based theory in an accessible and practical way. We hope this will enable veterinary healthcare teams to implement optimal interprofessional approaches to nutritional care and support for their individual situations. With its emphasis on collaborative working, this resource aims to be useful for all members of the veterinary healthcare team, including the clinical professions (veterinarians and veterinary nurses/technicians/assistants), other members of the practice team such as practice managers, those who work alongside practice teams (including animal industry representatives, such as nutritionists and dieticians), individuals interested in interprofessional education within undergraduate or postgraduate settings, and anyone studying veterinary medicine, veterinary nursing and animal care, and embarking on their future as a veterinary team member. Though written by professionals in the UK, we hope that the core messages from the book will also be relevant to veterinarians, vet techs and other allied professions and groups worldwide.

Before we begin, it is important to provide a definition of the term 'interprofessional' so that we can set expectations for readers of this book. Strictly speaking, this means 'between professionals'. The term 'professionals', of course, relates to members of a profession. But what is a profession? There are many ways to view the answer to this question, one being to consider a list of elements which makes a profession. A notable author in the area is Eliot Freidson, whose list of elements includes: a specific body of knowledge and skills, which leads to individuals with recognised credentials; division of labour being controlled by a working group, within a protected marketplace; in addition

DOI: 10.1079/9781800621107.0001

to an ideology of help over personal gain (Freidson, 2001). Veterinarians in the UK have long met this list of requirements, and more recently Registered Veterinary Nurses (RVNs) have done so as well, supported by the creation of a Register of RVNs and the proposal to protect the title. However, while much of this book will relate to these important veterinary professions, other groups and occupations which may not fit these strict criteria for a profession are no less important to our consideration of the veterinary team and will therefore be included. We believe that this focus on the interprofessional team is vital for providing the best possible care to our patients and clients, and is also of benefit to the teams themselves.

Several terms used within this book also require brief mention: veterinarian, veterinary nurse (VN), veterinary healthcare team (VHCT) and caretakers. These terms have been chosen to aid inclusivity and to reiterate the fact that the messages in this book are associated with more than simply 'veterinary surgeons' in the UK, 'veterinary techs' from the US, or individual pet caretakers and clients of a practice. The lessons we will explore for veterinary interprofessional teams can be developed from both human healthcare and aviation, where research into teamwork and the implications of different groups working together have been studied for many years. The similarities in the non-technical skills between aviation, human healthcare and veterinary care enable us to explore themes that have already been the subject of systematic study without reinventing the wheel. However, we must remember our own context, and that though similar, there are notable differences between working in an aeroplane cockpit, a rural (human medical) GP practice and an emergency room in a veterinary surgery! For example, Reeves *et al.* (2013) urged caution with simply using crew resource management (CRM) in other situations, and more recently Malcom *et al.* (2020) have reiterated the need for further research in human medicine, while also identifying transferable and useful aspects of CRM, such as a change in the way errors are managed, not avoided. Thus, while authors from human healthcare have looked to CRM for ideas, and while we will look to human medicine, it is also an aim of this book to share lessons learned from veterinary research into this complex topic as well as highlight the need for further context-based research.

This book aims to share, in an accessible way, some of the findings from interprofessional working, learning and education research, as well as experiences from professionals in the area of veterinary nutrition.

References

Freidson, E. (2001) *Professionalism: The Third Logic*. Polity Press, Cambridge, UK.
Malcom, D.R., Pate, A.N. and Rowe, A.S. (2020) Applying safety lessons from aviation to pre-licensure health professions education: A narrative critical review. *Currents in Pharmacy Teaching and Learning*, 12(8), 1028–1035.
Reeves, S., Kitto, S. and Masiello, I. (2013) Crew resource management: How well does it translate to an interprofessional healthcare context? *Journal of Interprofessional Care*, 27(3), 207–209.

Interprofessional working in veterinary practice

2

Tierney Kinnison

Abstract
There are many types of veterinary healthcare team (VHCT). VHCTs have developed over time, and now frequently include veterinarians and registered veterinary nurses, as well as other groups. The histories of these groups are vastly different; in the UK, veterinary nurses have been recognised, formally, as a profession since 2015, in stark contrast to the historic veterinary profession, whose professionalisation dates back to at least 1844. These historical differences lead to challenges in creating mutual understanding. Additional challenges to good working between these interprofessional groups include practicalities, attitudes and understanding of roles. However, when done well, there are many benefits to interprofessional working for patients, caretakers, the VHCT and veterinary practices. In this chapter, it is proposed that an awareness of regulatory body requirements and international developments in interprofessional competencies can help to guide understanding of necessary developments for creating optimal VHCTs which can work together on nutritional cases.

What is a veterinary healthcare team?

There is not a single correct answer to this question. It is likely that each reader of this chapter would answer the question in a different way, unique to their current situation and past experiences. It is also likely that the range of possible answers has changed over time.

Today, the composition of a veterinary healthcare team (VHCT) is rarely uni-professional, i.e. consisting of just one profession or occupation. However, historically, it may have been, or at least may have appeared so. A team can be multiprofessional, consisting of different professions or specialities, but working largely separately, for example within a referral hospital. Or it can be interprofessional, where the different professions and groups are working together for a common goal.

The goals of a VHCT may differ too, and may be focused on directly working with patients, developing education or practising research. Even if we

DOI: 10.1079/9781800621107.0002

consider just veterinary practices, the types of patients cared for, the caretakers seen, and the nature of the practice, be it corporate or independent, owned by a veterinarian or not, demonstrate a multivariable concept of veterinary healthcare goals.

Practically speaking, where the teams are located may differ; from large single-site practices to branch locations, to hub-and-satellite structures, and even extending to a partial or a purely online presence. In addition, personal aspects of the team may differ – a young team or older team, one which hosts students on placements or one that does not, and perhaps in the current era, an all-female team.

The literature has focused on several of these aspects which represent historic changes. For example, there has been a rise in the number of corporate practices, which has been a focus of research; a search of The Veterinary Record in PubMed shows the first mention of 'corporate' in 1985, followed by a gap of 11 years until a steady increase in publications from 1996 (one) to 2018 (five) with a drop in recent years. The feminisation of the veterinary profession is another area which has commanded much empirical research, as well as opinion pieces from the UK (Allen, 2016), the Netherlands (Koolmees, 2000) and the US (Smith, 2006), for example. There has, however, been relatively little research and conscious consideration of the changing interprofessional nature of the teams in which veterinary professions and occupations work, which has led to our current varied situation.

Throughout this book it is argued that this is an important research activity to conduct. It is suggested that understanding where we have come from and the experiences of our predecessors will assist with our interpretation of current interprofessional relationships, and potential ways forward, to implement optimal interprofessional approaches to care.

The development of the veterinary professions

At the start of my PhD, entitled 'Insights from Veterinary Interprofessional Interactions: Implications for Interprofessional Education (IPE) in the Veterinary Curricula' I wrote a paper with my supervisors on the rise of interprofessional practice within the veterinary field (Kinnison *et al.*, 2014). In this article we explored how researchers who have considered the development of veterinarians have typically done so in isolation from the other groups with which they have worked. In the article, we argued that it is important to consider the changing face of any single profession alongside those groups with which that profession works closely. After all, as one profession chooses to expand or contract its role (such as veterinarians moving from primarily working with equines and food animals towards primarily working with dogs and cats, and all the complexities this has brought about), other groups and professions fill in the gaps, or may potentially be required to give up their own roles.

The paper focuses on the professionalisation of the veterinary nurse (VN) in the UK. Consideration of the early stages of the veterinary nursing timeline has been collated by the Royal College of Veterinary Surgeons (RCVS) Knowledge Charitable Trust, and starts with the first RCVS approved Animal Nursing Auxiliary (ANA) training scheme in 1961 (RCVS Knowledge, n.d.). Since then, there have been a range of steps contributing to an overarching ability to recognise VNs as a profession at the time of publication of this book, including:

- inclusion of a list of VNs (2007) (now the Register)
- inclusion of disciplinary procedures (2011)
- a declaration of professional responsibilities (2012)
- requirement for continuing professional development for registered VNs (RVNs) (Kinnison *et al.*, 2014).

In 2015, a new supplemental Royal Charter was introduced, which confirmed the RCVS as the regulator of VNs, strengthened the Register of RVNs, and thus enhanced the accountability of RVNs for their own actions (RCVS, n.d.). These elements relate to Freidson's (2001) elements of a profession, as explored in the Introduction, and this Royal Charter demonstrates the continued commitment of the RCVS to veterinary nursing as a profession.

A further step for the development of this newer veterinary profession has been underway in bids to protect the title of 'veterinary nurse', so that only RVNs may use the term, and unqualified and unregistered laypeople may not refer to themselves by this name. In 2015, a petition was launched by the RCVS to the government to protect the title, and it received significant support from VNs alongside their colleagues from practice. However, the Department for Environment, Food & Rural Affairs (Defra) did not protect the title, claiming that the criminalisation for improper use of the title was unduly harsh (Woodmansey, 2016).

Since that time, the RCVS has set up another Legislation Working Party (LWP) (2017) to make recommendations for future veterinary legislation which have been reported and subjected to public consultation. The 'Recommendations for future veterinary legislation' (RCVS, 2021) calls for a new veterinary surgeons/services Act to replace the current 1966 Act, and incorporates veterinary professions and paraprofessions with the core focus on animal welfare and public protection. Notably, for VNs, the executive summary includes the following statements:

- 'By increasing opportunities for veterinary nurses and other allied professionals, the vision set out will create a more robust and flexible workforce and at the same time, increase efficiency within clinical practice.'
- 'Legislation should not be unduly burdensome or complicated; it should provide clarity to the public and enhance public confidence in the professions, e.g. protection of veterinary titles, statutory underpinning for continuing professional development (CPD).'

The recommendations also describe 'The vet-led team' (RCVS, 2021). This is a term which has been used to advocate for interprofessional working between veterinarians and other allied professions, and promotes a '"hub and spoke" model with the vet at the centre' (BVA, n.d.). However, the term and the model have not been received without confusion, for example regarding the regulation of the paraprofessions (Brizuela, 2019) and disappointment in relation to a lack of explicit inclusion of farriers (Dyer, 2019). In addition, it may be claimed that the portrayal of the veterinarian at the centre of the hub promotes the continuation of the hierarchical nature of veterinary practice, whereby the veterinarian maintains control of all the team's actions, potentially inhibiting the expertise of other groups, limiting their willingness to speak up and reducing efficiency in tasks where a veterinarian does not need to be directly involved. These aspects of interprofessional working are explored further in this book.

The existence of a veterinary hierarchy is not surprising when the differences in the history of the veterinarians and RVNs is examined. The history of RVNs as portrayed in this chapter is in stark contrast to that of veterinarians in the UK in terms of its timeframe, with veterinarians being recognised as a profession since the Royal Charter in 1844, compared to the date of 2015 cited above for RVNs. Being recognised as a profession was an early step in the development of veterinarians as we know them today, with further stages including the introduction of the first Veterinary Surgeons Act in 1881 and the updates in later years including in 1966, which together prevented unqualified practice and allowed only veterinarians to undertake and charge for acts of veterinary surgery (RCVS Knowledge, 2010).

The working relationship between veterinarians and RVNs is complex, not least of all because of the changes which the veterinary nursing profession is undergoing, which in turn have ramifications for the accountability of a VN. Although the RCVS legislation review (RCVS, 2021) considers removing the requirement for a VN to be employed by the veterinarian with whom they are working, 'under direction', it still mandates that VNs are working under the direction of veterinarians, who would usually be a part of the practice team in which they are employed, including their direct employers. Consequently, there is a complexity in the choices of VNs if presented with the requirement to undertake, or not undertake, action with which they disagree, potentially resulting in moral distress (Morley *et al.*, 2019), and even disciplinary procedures for the RVN. Further exploration of hierarchy and hierarchical interactions is found in Chapter 5.

Benefits of interprofessional teamworking

So why have RVNs risen as a profession, alongside other paraprofessional groups, including equine dentists, physiotherapists and animal behaviourists, to name but a few?

This chapter argues that the benefits of interprofessional working and a good team are obvious, with potential benefits for all stakeholders: the patients, the caretakers, the team and the practice.

A clear advantage for a team that integrates multiple professions, each with its own expertise, is that the team can benefit from the knowledge, skills and experience of all individuals, without requiring any one profession to know everything. This has been described as 'distributed' or 'team' cognition and is especially important for solving the complex problems (Hutchins, 1995; Salas *et al.*, 2007) that are common in medicine today, as our patients live longer and our understanding of diseases develops, and the demands of caretakers/our clients grows. For this to come to fruition, it can be seen that all professionals are required to recontextualise their knowledge (Guile, 2012). In essence, in order to share knowledge learned in their 'professional silos', in a way that is of use for the whole team and its members, within their new working environment, individuals adapt their understanding and see others' points of view in a way which is relevant to them. In a nice metaphor, this behaviour can be thought of as leading to a 'pool of shared meaning' (Patterson *et al.*, 2001) which is required in order for conversations to be effective and collective decisions to be able to be made. Ultimately, this can lead to 'collective competence', a useful term which reminds us that competence in a complex setting such as a veterinary practice is not only an individual trait, and that it is possible to have an incompetent team made up of competent individuals (Lingard, 2009).

At this point, to provide an overview of the research undertaken on the benefits of effective interprofessional teamworking, from micro to macro levels, the following are just a few examples from the literature on human and veterinary medicine outlining specific benefits of 'good' interprofessional working, i.e. collective competence, for the different stakeholder groups.

Benefits to:

- Patients: health
  - o a holistic view towards care with a focus on the patient (Walton *et al.*, 2019)
  - o reduction in medical error, contributed to by poor interprofessional behaviour including poor communication (Alvarez and Coiera, 2006; Kinnison *et al.*, 2015a, b).
- Patients: satisfaction (human healthcare, suggested as comparable to caretaker satisfaction in the veterinary field)
  - o increased patient satisfaction with collaborative care (Archer *et al.*, 2012).
- VHCT
  - o good collaboration and support (Horder, 2004).
- Practice
  - o economic advantages of using the correct profession for the appropriate roles (Getz, 2012).

In a case study of interprofessional working in the veterinary field, the following facilitators to interprofessional working which may lead to the aforementioned anticipated benefits were observed, and are considered further in this book (Kinnison *et al.*, 2016):

- different perspectives providing more holistic understanding of issues
- professionalisation and accountability of different groups involved
- hierarchy (appropriate)
- trust and value between all team members
- formal infrastructure that reinforces desired behaviours.

Challenges of interprofessional teamworking

It must be acknowledged that, like most examples of teamworking, there are many challenges to interprofessional working. A small selection of these, from the veterinary and human healthcare professions, are outlined below.

- Challenges:
  - time constraints (Walton *et al.*, 2019; Luebbers *et al.*, 2021)
  - coordination of teams (Walton *et al.*, 2019) including distributed teams due to physical location (Kinnison *et al.*, 2015a, b).
- Attitudes:
  - prejudice and lack of recognition, which can contribute to decisions to leave the profession (Robinson *et al.*, 2019)
  - inappropriate hierarchical behaviour when seeking advice and other resources (Kinnison *et al.*, 2016).
- Understanding:
  - lack of understanding of roles (Baxter and Brumfitt, 2008).

Direction for VHCT interprofessional working

The importance of overcoming these challenges and contributing to good interprofessional working has not been neglected within the global veterinary field and is highlighted within regulatory body requirements, for example, the RCVS's *Code of Professional Conduct for Veterinary Surgeons* includes the following professional responsibilities (RCVS, 2022b) which are mirrored in the *Code of Conduct for Veterinary Nurses* (RCVS, 2022a):

4. Veterinary surgeons and the veterinary team

4.1 Veterinary surgeons must work together and with others in the veterinary team and business, to co-ordinate the care of animals and the delivery of services.

4.2 Veterinary surgeons must ensure that tasks are delegated only to those who have the appropriate competence and registration.

4.3 Veterinary surgeons must maintain minimum practice standards equivalent to the Core Standards of the RCVS Practice Standards Scheme.

4.4 Veterinary surgeons must not impede professional colleagues seeking to comply with legislation and the RCVS Code of Professional Conduct.

4.5 Veterinary surgeons must communicate effectively, including in written and spoken English, with the veterinary team and other veterinary professionals in the UK.

In addition, within the veterinary code, there is advice and guidance relating how to work specifically with RVNs, in the section 'Delegation to veterinary nurses', which outlines the current Schedule 3 exemption (which allows nurses to legally practice), maintenance and monitoring of anaesthesia, vaccination of companion animals and dentistry.

The Interprofessional Education Collaborative has demonstrated four core competencies for interprofessional collaborative practice. While some edits are required for use in the veterinary field, these competencies are suggested to provide a useful starting point for consideration of improvements to interprofessional working.

- Competency 1: Work with individuals of other professions to maintain a climate of mutual respect and shared values. (Values/Ethics for Interprofessional Practice)
- Competency 2: Use the knowledge of one's own role and those of other professions to appropriately assess and address the health care needs of patients and to promote and advance the health of populations. (Roles/Responsibilities)
- Competency 3: Communicate with patients, families, communities, and professionals in health and other fields in a responsive and responsible manner that supports a team approach to the promotion and maintenance of health and the prevention and treatment of disease. (Interprofessional Communication)
- Competency 4: Apply relationship-building values and the principles of team dynamics to perform effectively in different team roles to plan, deliver, and evaluate patient/population centred care and population health programs and policies that are safe, timely, efficient, effective, and equitable. (Teams and Teamwork).

(Interprofessional Education Collaborative, 2016)

The penultimate chapter of this book will explore interprofessional education, which is proposed as a way to improve collaboration between professions, for the benefit of all stakeholders. In between this chapter and the penultimate chapter, we shall present evidence-based information regarding nutrition and the ability of VHCTs to achieve and maintain their place as the trusted and primary source of sound nutritional advice to animal caregivers.

In summary

Veterinary interprofessional teamwork in a VHCT can lead to many benefits for the different stakeholders but can be challenging to accomplish. Challenges to interprofessional working may stem in part from the historical differences in the two main veterinary professions (in the UK and, it is suggested, elsewhere), as well as the other occupations with which they work. There are ways for the VHCT to approach teamworking in order to optimise the approach taken, and these are explored in this book.

References

Allen, L.C.V. (2016) Feminisation: threat or opportunity? *Veterinary Record*, 178(16), 391–393.

Alvarez, G. and Coiera, E. (2006) Interdisciplinary communication: an uncharted source of medical error? *Journal of Critical Care*, 21(3), 236–242.

Archer, J., Bower, P., Gilbody, S., Lovell, K., Richards, D. *et al.* (2012) Collaborative care for depression and anxiety problems. *The Cochrane database of systematic reviews*. Available at: https://www.cochranelibrary.com/cdsr/doi/10.1002/14651858.CD006525.pub2/full (accessed 13 December 2022).

Baxter, S.K. and Brumfitt, S.M. (2008) Professional differences in interprofessional working. *Journal of Interprofessional Care*, 22, 239–251.

Brizuela, C. (2019) The vet-led team. *Veterinary Record*, 185(19), 602.

BVA (n.d.) The vet-led team. Available at: https://www.bva.co.uk/take-action/our-policies/the-vet-led-team/?dm_i=3VUQ%2CVL6G%2C1ZAMZW%2C378X6%2C1 (accessed 6 June 2022).

Dyer, H. (2019) The vet-led team. *Veterinary Record*, 185(19), 602.

Freidson, E. (2001) *Professionalism: The Third Logic*. Polity Press, Cambridge, UK.

Getz, M. (2012) Education and earnings in the health professions. *Journal of Veterinary Medical Education*, 39(3), 247–256.

Guile, D. (2012) Inter-professional working and learning: 'recontextualising' lessons from 'project work' for programmes of initial professional formation. *Journal of Education and Work*, 25(1), 79–99.

Horder, J. (2004) Interprofessional collaboration and interprofessional education. *The British Journal of General Practice: The Journal of the Royal College of General Practitioners*, 54(501), 243–245.

Hutchins, E. (1995) *Cognition in the Wild*. MIT Press, Cambridge, UK.

Interprofessional Educational Collaborative (2016) Core competencies for inter-professional collaborative practice: 2016 update. Available at: https://ipec.memberclicks.net/assets/2016-Update.pdf (accessed 13 December 2022).

Kinnison, T., May, S.A. and Guile, D. (2014) Inter-professional practice: from vet-erinarian to the veterinary team. *Journal of Veterinary Medical Education*, 41(2), 172–178.

Kinnison, T., Guile, D. and May, S.A. (2015a) Errors in veterinary practice: prelim-inary lessons for building better veterinary teams. *The Veterinary Record*, 177(19), 492.

Kinnison, T., May, S.A. and Guile, D. (2015b) Veterinary team interactions, part one: The practice effect. *Veterinary Record*, 177(16), 419.

Kinnison, T., Guile, D. and May, S.A. (2016) The case of veterinary interprofessional practice: From one health to a world of its own. *Journal of Interprofessional Education and Practice*, 4, 51–57.

Koolmees, P.A. (2000) Feminization of veterinary medicine in the Netherlands 1925–2000. *Argos*, 23, 125–131.

Lingard, L. (2009) What we see and don't see when we look at 'competence': Notes on a god term. *Advances in Health Sciences Education*, 14(5), 625–628.

Luebbers, J., Gurenlian, J. and Freudenthal, J. (2021) Physicians' perceptions of the role of the dental hygienist in interprofessional collaboration: a pilot study. *Journal of Interprofessional Care*, 35(1), 132–135.

Morley, G., Ives, J., Bradbury-Jones, C. and Irvine, F. (2019) What is 'moral distress'? A narrative synthesis of the literature. *Nursing Ethics*, 26(3), 646–662.

Patterson, K., Grenny, J., McMillan, R. and Switzler, A. (2001) *Crucial conversations: Tools for talking when stakes are high*. McGraw-Hill, New York, USA.

RCVS (2021) Recommendations for future veterinary legislation. Available at: https://www.rcvs.org.uk/news-and-views/publications/rcvs-recommendations-for-future-veterinary-legislation/ (accessed 13 December 2022).

RCVS (2022a) *Code of Conduct for Veterinary Nurses*. Available at: https://www.rcvs.org.uk/setting-standards/advice-and-guidance/code-of-professional-conduct-for-veterinary-nurses/#team (accessed 23 May 2022).

RCVS (2022b) *Code of Professional Conduct for Veterinary Surgeons*. Available at: https://www.rcvs.org.uk/setting-standards/advice-and-guidance/code-of-professional-conduct-for-veterinary-surgeons/#team (accessed 23 May 2022).

RCVS (n.d.) About the VN Register. Available at: https://www.rcvs.org.uk/registration/check-the-register/about-the-vn-register/ (accessed 23 May 2022).

RCVS Knowledge (2010) British veterinary medicine timeline. Available at: https://knowledge.rcvs.org.uk/heritage-and-history/history-of-the-veterinary-profession/british-veterinary-medicine-timeline/ (accessed 6 June 2022).

RCVS Knowledge (n.d.) Veterinary nursing timeline. Available at: http://knowledge.rcvs.org.uk/heritage-and-history/history-of-the-veterinary-profession/veterinary-nursing-timeline/ (accessed 21 September 2015).

Robinson, D., Edwards, M., Akehurst, G., Cockett, J. *et al.* (2019) The 2019 Survey of the Veterinary Nurse Profession. Available at: https://www.rcvs.org.uk/news-and-views/publications/the-2019-survey-of-the-veterinary-nursing-profession/ (accessed 13 December 2022).

Salas, E., Rosen, M.A., Burke, C.S., Nicholson, D. and Howse, W.R. (2007) Markers for Enhancing Team Cognition in Complex Environments: The Power of Team Performance Diagnosis. *Aviation, Space, and Environmental Medicine*, 78(5 Suppl), B77–85.

Smith, C.A. (2006) The gender shift in veterinary medicine: Cause and effect. *Veterinary Clinics of North America – Small Animal Practice*, 36(2), 329–339.

Walton, V., Hogden, A., Long, J.C., Johnson, J.K. and Greenfield, D. (2019) How do interprofessional healthcare teams perceive the benefits and challenges of interdisciplinary ward rounds? *Journal of Multidisciplinary Healthcare*, 12, 1023–1032.

Woodmansey, D. (2016) Setback for campaign to protect 'veterinary nurse' title. *The Veterinary Times*. Available at: https://www.vettimes.co.uk/news/setback-for-campaign-to-protect-veterinary-nurse-title/ (accessed 6 June 2022).

Optimising pet health and wellbeing through nutrition

3

Rachel Lumbis

Abstract

Correct nutrition is a key factor in optimising animal health, wellbeing, performance and quality of life, but considerable confusion, widespread myths and misinformation exist regarding nutritional facts and dietary choices. Not all sources of pet nutrition information are equal, therefore it is a responsibility of the veterinary healthcare team (VHCT) to be a trusted and primary source of sound nutritional advice and to signpost clients to appropriate dietary resources. Feeding is a daily interaction between clients and their pets, and many caretakers gain great satisfaction and enjoyment from watching their pets eat. Educating about suitable feeding protocols and diet choice can help to preserve the bond between pets and caretakers. The humanisation of animals is driving expansion of the pet food market, yet anthropomorphism can result in inappropriate food-related behaviours, compromising nutritional welfare. This chapter will consider feeding as a fundamental responsibility of pet caretakers, highlight the importance of optimal pet nutrition to health, wellbeing and longevity, outline sources of nutrition information and identify ways of evaluating information quality.

The importance of optimal pet nutrition

Optimal nutrition is a cornerstone for health and is fundamental to wellbeing, longevity, and disease prevention and management. Defined as the process of providing and obtaining the food necessary for health and growth (Arai, 2014), the importance of nutrition has been recognised for over 2000 years since the time of Hippocrates. The body is in a continual state of hunger, which is intermittently relieved by eating. This perpetual drive to eat is periodically suppressed by inhibitory impulses generated by factors including presence of food in the gastrointestinal tract and the flow of nutrients into blood. After these satiety factors have dissipated, the desire to eat returns. A limited or excessive appetite is not necessarily pathological. Both genetic and environmental factors may regulate appetite, and abnormalities in either may lead to abnormal appetite. Abnormal appetite could be defined as eating habits

© Rachel Lumbis and Tierney Kinnison 2023. *An Interprofessional Approach to Veterinary Nutrition* (R. Lumbis and T. Kinnison)
DOI: 10.1079/9781800621107.0003

causing malnutrition and related conditions such as obesity and its associated problems. Factors that affect normal intake of food include:

- sensory factors
- psychological factors
- environmental factors
- physical factors
- age/life stage.

The primary role of diet is to provide sufficient nutrients and energy to meet metabolic requirements while giving the consumer a feeling of wellbeing (Bontempo, 2005). Appropriate feeding protocols and diet choice plays a critical role in the care and clinical outcome of healthy and clinically affected companion animals (Carciofi and Brunetto, 2009), contributing to:

- extension of life expectancy in dogs (Kealy *et al.*, 2002)
- improved response to trauma and stress (Kathrani, 2016)
- more rapid recovery (Mohr *et al.*, 2003; Sallander and Jaktlund, 2012/2013; Mansfield and Beths, 2015)
- preservation of lean body mass (Kathrani, 2016)
- better hospital and patient outcomes (Remillard *et al.*, 2001; Brunetto *et al.*, 2010; Harris *et al.*, 2017)
- shorter time to discharge (Brunetto *et al.*, 2010; Liu *et al.*, 2012)
- decreased mortality (Chan *et al.*, 2002) and morbidity (Kathrani, 2016).

Three main components influence the life of an animal: genetics, the environment and nutrition. Of these, nutrition is the single factor that veterinary professionals can influence to maximise health, improve performance and longevity, and manage disease (Burns, 2014). The global rise of diet-related non-communicable diseases and increase in the popularity of alternative and unconventional diets means it is imperative that the VHCT can provide, at minimum, fundamental nutrition advice based on sound scientific evidence.

Human–animal interaction

Human–animal interactions are very diverse and, over the years, strong emotional connections with animals have been formed through their use as pets and companions; for sport and recreation; animal husbandry; and in animal-assisted therapies. Increasing human–animal interaction has led to domestication through anthropomorphism and the ascribing of human predilections and characteristics to animals, with many pets now considered quasi-human (Fig. 3.1). Culture also influences the degree to which people project human mental states on other species (Epley *et al.*, 2007).

The degree of attachment between people and animals varies and relationships can be situational and conditional, depending on how animals are viewed (Amiot *et al.*, 2016). The term 'human–animal bond' (HAB) was coined in

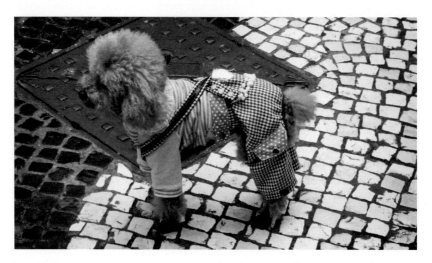

Fig. 3.1. Dressing up pets is an example of anthropomorphism. Despite the associated welfare issues, for some caretakers this practice is a light-hearted way of demonstrating their affection for their pet, reinforcing the human–animal bond. Photograph: author.

1977 and is now also known as 'human–companion animal bond' (Solhjoo *et al.*, 2018). According to the Human Animal Bond Research Institute (HABRI, 2022), the human–animal bond (HAB) is a 'mutually beneficial and dynamic relationship between people and animals that is influenced by behaviours that are essential to the health and well-being of both. This includes, but is not limited to, emotional, psychological, and physical interactions of people, animals, and the environment.'

The post-World War II years saw an increase in pet ownership and changes in the importance of, and human interaction with, companion animals (Herzog, 2014). Pet-keeping is common in many, if not most, human societies (Herzog, 2014); an estimated half of all households worldwide include an animal (Westgarth *et al.*, 2010) with younger generations making up 50% of all pet owners. The coronavirus pandemic saw an increased demand for pets, and pet ownership surged by around 20% in most of the developed world. This was especially prevalent among new and inexperienced owners, with many from the younger generations, Z and millennial, aged between 16 and 34 years (Wedderburn, 2022). Although the number and species of animals kept as pets varies across countries and cultures, dogs and cats are among the most popular (Wanser *et al.*, 2019). Recognition and engagement with the HAB have driven a change in terminology and regard of companion animals as 'pets', 'family members', 'fur-babies', 'fur-kids' and 'boys and girls' (Wedderburn, 2022). The term 'owner' is now seen to infer pets as property, rather than living creatures. This viewpoint represents only 1% of pet owners (Boss *et al.*, 2021) and fails to accurately reflect pet-keeping in modern society, therefore use of the term 'pet parent' is becoming more common. For the purposes of this publication, the term 'caretaker' is used throughout to denote pet owners and individuals with responsibility for the care and wellbeing of a companion animal.

The HAB can generate widespread positive sentiment towards animals, contribute to increases in the life expectancy of pet dogs and cats and influence expected level of care. A high proportion of pet caretakers consider their animals as family members or companions and actively seek for them a long and healthy life (Cohen, 2002; Bontempo, 2005; Carlisle-Frank and Frank, 2006; Boss *et al.*, 2021). Clients who understand that preventative care preserves and lengthens their relationship with their pets are more likely to use veterinary services regularly. Hence, the HAB is extremely important to most clients of small animal veterinary practices (Friedmann and Son, 2009), with a stronger pet–caretaker bond associated with a higher level of expected care (Lue *et al.*, 2008). As highlighted by Johnson (2022), it is therefore essential for the VHCT to acknowledge and integrate the HAB into clinical culture to ensure provision of the highest quality patient care (Fig. 3.2).

Pets are often an important part of their caretakers' lives and are associated with the alleviation of stress and improvement of mental wellbeing (PDSA, 2021) among many other social and physiological health benefits identified by FEDIAF (2022a). These include:

- decreased blood pressure with a lower incidence of cardiovascular disease
- reduced risk of mortality
- decreased cholesterol levels
- decreased triglyceride levels
- positive contribution to health and wellbeing
- increased opportunities for exercise and outdoor activities
- reduced feelings of loneliness and social isolation
- increased opportunities for socialisation.

These benefits are also linked to the quality of the bond, not merely due to the presence of a pet in the household. In children, a strong child–animal bond

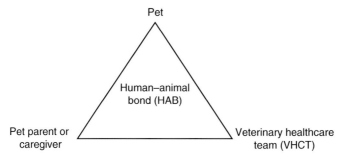

Fig. 3.2. The HAB is at the centre of the veterinary health triangle, all components of which can benefit from each other. To optimise the provision of veterinary care, the VHCT should leverage the HAB, placing it at the centre of client communication. Author's own figure.

(Fig. 3.3) can produce several positive effects in physiological, cognitive and socio-emotional development, including:

- decreased blood pressure and heart rate (Wanser *et al.*, 2019)
- increased likelihood of being physically active (children from dog-owning households) (Gadomski *et al.*, 2017)
- a reduction in children's pain perception, fatigue, distress, fear and sadness and a more rapid recovery time in hospital settings (McCullough *et al.*, 2018)
- facilitation of learning, contributing to educational and life success (Gee *et al.*, 2017)
- improvements in sense of confidence (Gee *et al.*, 2017)
- development of empathy, kindness and concern for others (Poresky, 1990; Vidović *et al.*, 1999)
- stronger pro-social orientations (Vidović *et al.*, 1999; Gee *et al.*, 2019)
- assumption of a caretaker role and learning responsibility (Fifield and Forsyth, 1999).

Pets provide both an opportunity for caretakers to receive emotional support from a non-judgemental individual, and to express caregiving behaviours in return (Fig. 3.4). Being expressions of empathy, both the giving and receiving of care provide similar positive emotional benefits to people, with the provision and consumption of food considered primary means of human expression of care (Hamburg *et al.*, 2014) (Fig. 3.5). Those who are out of the house for long periods each day may regard feeding as a main point of contact with their pet.

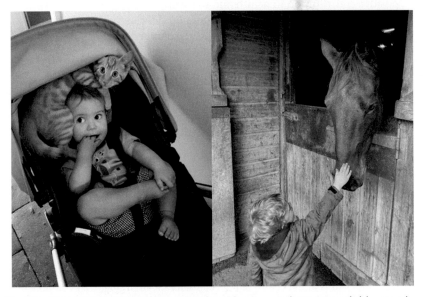

Fig. 3.3. Pet attachment is a fundamental mechanism underpinning child–animal interactions and relationships, with a strong bond associated with a higher quality of life and positive future behaviour towards animals. Photograph: author.

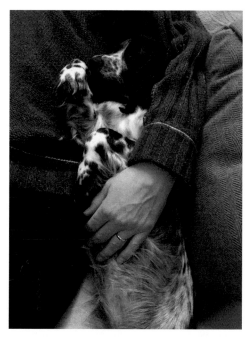

Fig. 3.4. Pets are often an important part of their caretakers' lives, and it is important that the VHCT leverages this bond when communicating about nutrition. Photograph: author.

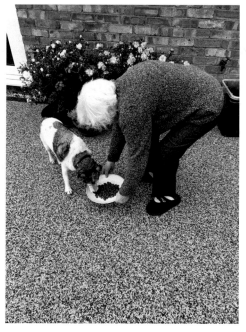

Fig. 3.5. For some caretakers, offering food to a pet and seeing it eaten are important aspects of expressing care, with affection or love for an animal most pronounced through the provision of food. Photograph: author.

Maintaining the health of pets through the provision of correct nutrition is an essential component of being a responsible pet caretaker and one that caretakers are becoming increasingly aware of as a key factor in optimising pet health and wellbeing. Educating about appropriate feeding protocols and diet choice helps to preserve the bond between pets and caretakers, therefore the VHCT should focus on proper nutrition for every patient that presents to their practice.

Feeding as a fundamental part of responsible ownership and the influence of cognitive bias

Nutrition is integral to optimal animal care with an ultimate goal to feed for ideal health, performance and longevity. Prior to domestication, dogs and cats were primarily kept as working animals, living outside and being fed raw meat or table scraps. The humanisation of animals and current-day notion of pets as family members is a key trend which, together with numerous developments in companion animal nutrition, is driving the pet food market (FEDIAF, 2022b). Consequently, a wide array of pet food is now available with a rise in the availability of conventional and unconventional diets, and the growing popularity of unconventional 'fad' pet foods (home-cooked, raw, grain-free, vegetarian, vegan) and innovative diets (novel protein-based). Europe is considered an industry leader, generating around 30% of the total pet food and pet care sales, worldwide (FEDIAF, 2022b). The UK pet food market is worth a total of £3.3 billion (PFMA, 2022).

With the current availability of such a broad range of pet foods, caretakers can select the food they believe to be most appropriate for their pet. Factors influencing pet food selection and purchase include personal circumstances and biases, 'gut feelings', cultural identity, past experiences, flavour preferences and dietary predilections, in addition to ingredients, quality, cost, manufacturer's reputation, veterinary recommendation and ease of purchasing (Simonsen et al., 2014; Conway and Saker, 2018; Schleicher et al., 2019). The influence of cognitive bias in dietary decision-making is significant, particularly the Dunning-Kruger effect whereby individuals with limited or no knowledge, skill and expertise overestimate their own cognitive ability and competence (Chandler, 2018). When presented with information, even irrefutable evidence, people still gravitate towards sources most closely aligned with their own views and beliefs, even if these are inaccurate and misinformed, and refute any opposing ideas or theories. This must be considered when communicating with pet caretakers about nutritional facts and dietary choices and is discussed further in Chapter 7.

Many caretakers award greater consideration to their pet's diet than their own, with over half giving equal or more priority to buying healthy food for their pets compared with themselves (Schleicher et al., 2019). Yet when translated into human behaviour and actions, this has the potential to benefit and compromise the nutritional welfare of pets. In human medicine, poor diet is the second leading cause of death in the world (Adamski et al.,

2018). The anthropomorphic nature of many human–companion animal relationships, combined with considerable confusion and misinformation about human and pet nutrition, can result in inappropriate food-related behaviours and the feeding of suboptimal, or even dangerous, diets, with deleterious effects on health and wellbeing (Wensley, 2008). The use of terms such as 'premium', 'super-premium', 'natural', 'hypoallergenic' and 'holistic' can often prove appealing, yet are unregulated and promote product sales rather than indicate nutritional quality. Other marketing strategies and health claims, combined with caretaker inability to accurately interpret pet food labels (Sapowicz *et al.*, 2016; Yam *et al.*, 2017) can make appropriate pet food selection challenging, with many caretakers finding this the most difficult aspect of pet ownership (Schleicher *et al.*, 2019).

Diet is one aspect of pet welfare that has been notably affected by the COVID-19 outbreak. In the UK, over 1.4 million pets have reportedly gained weight since the start of the pandemic, with increases in treat-giving and a larger provision of human food as part of pets' main meals, contributing to the rise in canine and feline obesity diagnosis and the existing pet obesity crisis (Evason *et al.*, 2020; PDSA, 2021). Similar findings have been identified in the US (Pet Food Industry, 2020). Obesity is a modern-day epidemic in both people and companion animals (Kipperman and German, 2018) and is considered present in the latter when ideal bodyweight is exceeded by 30% or more (Ward *et al.*, 2019). It is a disease of rapidly increasing prevalence in dogs and cats and is considered the biggest current health and welfare concern for companion animals in developed countries (Sandøe *et al.*, 2014). The problem is exacerbated by:

- pet caretakers' lack of awareness of their pet's body condition score and body weight, and an inability to recognise if these are appropriate or not (Yam *et al.*, 2017; Evason *et al.*, 2020)
- the normalisation of excess weight, with a higher body condition considered optimal (Evason *et al.*, 2020)
- pet caretakers' failure to view excessive weight as a concern within the context of animal health (Wainwright *et al.*, 2022)
- not following or understanding pet food feeding guidelines (BVA, 2016; Yam *et al.*, 2017)
- excessive treat and food provision (BVA, 2016)
- insufficient exercise provision (BVA, 2016)
- obesity being a frustratingly difficult condition to reverse, with weight loss proving challenging to maintain (Larsen and Villaverde, 2016).

It is therefore critical that the VHCT is confident in educating pet caretakers and is viewed as the primary and trusted source of nutritional advice.

Sources of nutrition information

Today's pet caretakers are informed consumers (Boss *et al.*, 2021) with the ability to access a wide range of nutrition-related advice and information sources, and with preferences for how, and from whom, this is delivered. Pet caretakers' engagement with the recommendations of veterinary professionals varies with some actively seeking advice, others willing to accept advice but reluctant to ask for it, through to those who are sceptical of veterinary advice and choose to avoid and/or ignore this (Chandler, 2018). Yet many caretakers look to veterinary professionals to provide advice on optimal nutrition, appropriate to the species, life stage and health status of pets. It is essential for the VHCT to ensure the HAB is translated into optimal caretaker dietary choices and feeding practices, conductive to good nutritional welfare, by providing sound and fundamental nutritional advice throughout each stage of a pet's life. The veterinary consultation is identified as a foremost client contact point for nutritional discussion (Lumbis and de Scally, 2020), yet while a reported 57–90% of pet caretakers believe a nutritional recommendation from the VHCT to be important (AAHA, 2003; Flocke *et al.*, 2013; Evason *et al.*, 2020), only 15–23% perceive they have received one (AAHA, 2003; Flocke *et al.*, 2013; Morgan *et al.*, 2017). Nutritional interventions are not being translated into the training or practice of practitioners (Becvarova *et al.*, 2016). Consequently, nutrition is infrequently discussed during healthy and sick pet appointments (Bergler *et al.*, 2016; Morgan *et al.*, 2017; Evason *et al.*, 2020; Alvarez *et al.*, 2022) and complete nutritional assessments are scarcely performed during veterinary consultations (Bergler *et al.*, 2016; Bruckner and Handl, 2020; Lumbis and de Scally, 2020). Potential reasons for this are explored in Chapter 4, with proposed resolutions provided in subsequent chapters.

While the VHCT is considered a leading authority and trusted information source on pet nutrition and healthcare, (Kienzle *et al.*, 1998; Michel *et al.*, 2008; Connolly *et al.*, 2014; Schleicher *et al.*, 2019; Lai et al., 2021) there is a growing distrust in the nutritional advice provided by the VHCT and preferred use of alternative sources (Schleicher *et al.*, 2019), particularly among select caretaker demographics. Less than half of dog breeders ask their veterinarian for nutritional advice (Connolly *et al.*, 2014). Evidence further suggests that pet caretakers feeding raw and non-commercial diets have limited trust in veterinarians' ability to provide sound nutritional advice, relying more on their own knowledge (Empert-Gallegos *et al.*, 2020) and online resources (Michel *et al.*, 2008; Connolly *et al.*, 2014).

Many caretakers consider the internet a favoured (Kogan *et al.*, 2018; Wainwright *et al.*, 2022) or complimentary (Solhjoo *et al.*, 2017) source of information to the VHCT. As a core pillar of the modern information society, the internet and social media has a global penetration rate of 63 and 59% respectively, equating to around 5 billion users worldwide (Statista, 2022). With continued expansion of the internet and nearly two thirds of the global population now connected to the World Wide Web, there is a large abundance of information at users' disposal and its influence is growing. People are assuming more active roles in making healthcare decisions for themselves and family members (Kogan et al., 2012), the latter of which is now commonly extended to include pets (Wedderburn, 2022). In human medicine, the internet is a widely and commonly used source for health information, helping to empower and inform patients (Kogan *et al.*, 2010, 2012; Kuhl *et al.*, 2022), improve the patient–practitioner relationship and enhance the consultation experience through more effective communication (Boden, 2018). It is also increasingly becoming the first point of contact for pet caretakers seeking advice about the health and welfare of their animal and to help educate and guide them in making informed decisions about their pet's wellbeing, care and treatment (Murphy, 2006; Kogan *et al.*, 2014; Kuhl *et al.*, 2022).

The availability of online information about pet nutrition and diet is substantial and it is one of the most frequently searched topics by pet caretakers (Kogan *et al.*, 2010; Kogan *et al.*, 2018; Kuhl *et al.*, 2022). A Google search using the words '[pet nutrition information]' in May 2022 resulted in 198,000,000 hits. Other pet health information sources include past experience and own knowledge; friends, family and colleagues; social media and online forums; animal shelters, rescues and charities; breeders; pet shops; magazines, newspapers and books. Several factors, including convenience, trustworthiness and the HAB, are considered to influence and affect pet caretakers' choice of information source and information search behaviour (Holbrook 1996; Lancendorfer *et al.*, 2008). Caretakers with a strong attachment to their pets seek active participation in the information search process, favouring communication channels that are informational or need to be actively searched, such as print media or the internet. Those with reduced attachment to their pets prefer passive receipt of information and demonstrate more reliance on broadcast media, such as television and radio.

Evaluating information quality

Information sources, particularly those obtained through the internet and social media, can positively and negatively influence caretakers' decision-making and, thus, the health and welfare of their pets (Kogan *et al.*, 2019, 2021; Kuhl *et al.*, 2022). The proliferation of available information, absence of reliable indicators of resource quality and lack of enforced system for quality control online (Kuhl *et al.*, 2022), combined with caretakers' preference for the use of search engines over direct access to specific pet health websites (Kogan *et al.*, 2010), means navigating the internet can be challenging (Boden, 2018) and overwhelming. Anyone can post data and information on the internet, promoting themselves as experts. Consequently, the quality of online information varies and can often be anecdotal or opinion-based with no scientific grounding. Few pet caretakers have the desire or ability to assess the reliability, accuracy and credibility of information (Kogan *et al.*, 2012; Solhjoo *et al.*, 2018) or to understand and interpret this (Kogan *et al.*, 2010; Kogan and Oxley, 2020), resulting in low health literacy with potential confusion, misinformation, conflicting messaging and a negative impact on the relationship between clients and the VHCT (Kogan and Oxley, 2020). Yet confidence in information obtained from veterinary professionals remains high (Kogan *et al.*, 2010; Kuhl *et al.*, 2022).

Guidance relating to effective use of the internet to search for veterinary/ pet health information is limited (Kogan *et al.*, 2010) and is identified as a concern by veterinarians (Boden, 2018), yet few veterinary practices supply pet health website information or veterinarian-recommended websites to their clients (Kogan *et al.*, 2018; Kogan and Oxley, 2020). It is essential for the VHCT to assume a proactive role in raising awareness of the quality of pet health information online and to consider providing 'information prescriptions' to guide the information-seeking behaviours of pet caretakers (Solhjoo *et al.*, 2018; Kogan and Oxley, 2020). Signposting clients towards credible, valid, accurate and trustworthy online information sources (Table 3.1) provides an adjunct form of client education that can enhance the information provided by veterinary professionals (Kogan *et al.*, 2012). It also facilitates better, evidence-based pet dietary decision-making by caretakers (Oxley *et al.*, 2017; Kogan *et al.*, 2018) and enhanced communication with veterinary professionals (Kogan *et al.*, 2014), ultimately, benefiting all parties (Kogan *et al.*, 2008).

A well-known strategy used to evaluate the quality of online (and offline) information sources is the CRAAP (currency, relevance, authority, accuracy, purpose) test (California State University, 2010). This method prompts consideration of these five criteria through the completion of a variety of questions, examples of which are included in Table 3.2. The level of importance placed on each evaluation criteria will vary according to individual situation or need. While the method is not without its limitations, it can be a useful evaluation tool for the VHCT and pet caretakers to use when assessing information sources on different aspects of pet care, including nutrition.

Additional considerations and checks proposed by the WSAVA (2013a, b) include the following.

- **Identification of the website's domain**
  Consider the website name, its logo, the URL of the website (Table 3.3), the internet address and other indicators that can help to prove its reliability on the topic. Is the website reputable and credible on the subject matter? Can it be considered an authority site for factual information? How often does the website publish content and related content? Large pet food companies often have high quality information that is separate from their product information.
- **Be sceptical of grand claims or easy answers to difficult questions**
  It is easy, though illegal, to make unproven claims for nutritional products but it is much harder to provide scientific backing. If it sounds too good to be true, it probably is.
- **Watch out for rating websites**
  Most websites that rank pet food do so either on opinion or using subjective criteria that do not necessarily ensure a good quality food (e.g., price, ingredients, company size). More objective criteria should be used, including scientific substantiation and quality control.

Table 3.1. Useful and accurate online sources of veterinary nutrition information.

Nutritional assessment and associated tools

World Small Animal Veterinary Association (WSAVA) Global Nutrition Toolkit https://WSAVA-Global-Nutrition-Toolkit-English.pdf	Freely available, non-branded practical aids to make nutrition assessment and recommendations more efficient, as well as educational materials for pet caretakers. You can also download a copy of the WSAVA Nutritional Assessment Guidelines from here.
World Small Animal Veterinary Association (WSAVA) Nutrition Assessment Guidelines https://wsava.org/Global-Guidelines/Global-Nutrition-Guidelines/	A direct link to the WSAVA Nutritional Assessment Guidelines.
Pet Nutrition Alliance https://petnutritionalliance.org/	A variety of educational materials and tools for pet caretakers and the VHCT, including tips for implementing nutrition as a vital assessment in practice.

FAQs and general nutrition information for pet owners and/or the VHCT

Association of American Feed Control Officials (AAFCO) https://www.aafco.org/	Sets standards for the quality and safety of animal feed and pet food in the US. Produces guidance on topics including nutrient and dietary requirements and labelling.
American Veterinary Medical Association (AVMA) https://www.avma.org/resources/pet-owners/petcare/getting-pet-health-information-online	Information to assist pet caretakers in identifying reliable pet health information online.
British Small Animal Veterinary Association (BSAVA) Guide to Nutrition (and factsheets) https://www.bsavalibrary.com/content/book/10.22233/9781910443828#overview	This guide offers information on commercially manufactured diets, grain-free diets, home-prepared cooked diets and raw diets, together with a range of veterinary and pet caretaker factsheets. Access is subject to a fee.
Clinical Nutrition Service at Cummings School of Veterinary Medicine, Tufts University https://vetnutrition.tufts.edu/petfoodology/	The answers to several frequently asked client questions are available here including general pet nutrition advice, home-cooked diets for pets and information on the care and use of feeding tubes at home.

Continued

Table 3.1. Continued.

Fédération Européenne De l'industrie des aliments pour animaux Familiers (FEDIAF) (European Pet Food Industry) https://www.fediaf.org	Guidelines and factsheets on a range of topics relevant to the pet food industry in Europe. These include nutrient and dietary requirements; pet food facts; legislation, labelling, quality and safety of pet food; responsible pet ownership; and environment and sustainability.
Global Alliance of Pet Food Associations (GAPFA) https://www.gapfa.org/library	A range of educational information and factsheets about the global pet food industry, pet food safety, dog and cat nutrition and responsible pet ownership.
National Research Council of the National Academies (NRC) 1. https://nap.nationalacademies.org/resource/10668/cat_nutrition_final.pdf 2. https://nap.nationalacademies.org/resource/10668/dog_nutrition_final_fix.pdf	A science-based guide for pet caretakers on a cat's nutritional needs (1) and a dog's nutritional needs (2).
Nutrologia de cães e gatos https://nutrologiadecaesegatos.com.br/	Based in Brazil, 'The dog and cat nutrology blog' highlights the importance of quality food for the good health and wellbeing of pets.
Pet Obesity Prevention https://petobesityprevention.org/	Tools and information on weight reduction to help the VHCT and pet caretakers to assess body condition, ideal body weight, calorie requirements and optimal weight loss.
UK Pet Food (formerly known as the Pet Food Manufacturers' Association or PFMA) https://www.ukpetfood.org/	Supports dynamic and responsible UK pet food manufacturing and provides educational information on pet nutrition and the manufacture of pet food. Also, commissions new research into the UK's pet population and provides useful relevant statistics.
Vet Specialists – Board-Certified veterinary experts https://www.vetspecialists.com/specialties/nutrition	Information for pet caretakers about Board-Certified Veterinary Nutritionists, pet food, feeding management and clinical conditions.

Continuing education (CE)/continuing professional development (CPD)

There is a wide range of CE and CPD available, online and in-person, and it is beyond the scope of this publication to provide a comprehensive list of worldwide providers. Readers are encouraged to review the local CPD courses and conferences presented by universities, veterinary professional associations, regulatory bodies and accredited service providers in their own country.

Academy of Veterinary Nutrition Technicians (AVNT)
http://nutritiontechs.org/

Developing the knowledge and expertise of veterinary technicians/nurses and endorsing them as a vital part of the veterinary nutrition profession. Here you will find information on the Veterinary Technician Speciality (VTS) nutrition course as well as links to other nutrition-related resources.

American College of Veterinary Internal Medicine (ACVIM)
https://www.acvim.org/resources-for

The home of ACVIM specialists, including Board-Certified Veterinary Nutritionists, a variety of resources are available, aimed at a range of groups including pet caretakers, diplomates, primary care veterinarians, VNs and students.

British Small Animal Veterinary Association (BSAVA)
https://www.bsava.com/education/cpd/

BSAVA offers a vast range of online and in-person veterinary CPD, covering clinical and non-clinical topics.

The Webinar Vet
https://www.thewebinarvet.com/

Online CPD available live and on demand, covering a wide range of topics across large and small animal species, suitable for the VHCT.

Vetacademy
https://vetacademy.org/

Vetacademy covers all aspects of veterinary practice: clinical (companion animal and livestock); management and leadership; customer service; soft skills; and communication. Content is suitable for veterinarians, veterinary nurses (VNs)/technicians, managers, receptionists and support staff.

Vetlexicon
https://www.vetlexicon.com/

A veterinary clinical reference source, providing peer-reviewed and evidence-based information, images, videos and client factsheets on a wide range of species and topics. Access is subject to a fee.

Continued

Table 3.1. Continued.

WikiVet https://en.wikivet.net/Veterinary_Education_Online	A free veterinary encyclopedia. WikiVet is a worldwide collaborative project to develop a comprehensive online peer-reviewed veterinary knowledge database that aims to cover the entire undergraduate curriculum.
World Small Animal Veterinary Association (WSAVA) Academy https://academy-wsava.thinkific.com/	The WSAVA Academy features lectures and courses, covering both clinical and practice management topics to support all members of the VHCT. Among the available content is a four-module course on the key aspects of the WSAVA Global Nutrition Guidelines which can be accessed without charge: https://academy-wsava.thinkific.com/courses/nutrition-guidelines
Veterinary nutritionists	
American College of Veterinary Internal Medicine (Nutrition) diplomates https://www.vetspecialists.com	The online directory that allows you to search for Board-Certified Veterinary Nutritionists of the American College of Veterinary Internal Medicine (ACVIM).
European College of Veterinary and Comparative Nutrition (ECVCN) https://ebvs.eu/colleges/ECVCN	A link to the Diplomate Directory to locate an EBVS (European Board of Veterinary Specialisation) European Specialist in Veterinary and Comparative Nutrition.

Table 3.2. An adaptation of the CRAAP test, originally created by Sarah Blakeslee of the Meriam Library at the California State University and reproduced with permission. This method uses five verification steps to check the objective reliability and credibility of online and offline information sources.

Currency – the timeliness of the information

- Is the information up to date? When was the information published/posted?
- Has the web page/information been updated or modified recently? If so, cross check the published information to ascertain its currency.
- Are the sources/citations used by the author(s) current or outdated?
- Are appropriate web links supplied? If so, are these functional?

Relevance – the appropriateness of the information

- Is the information directly related to your topic of interest/context/research question?
- Who is the intended readership or audience?
- Is it appropriate in terms of academic level? Is it too simple/elementary or too advanced/complex?
- Have other sources of information been considered in addition to, or instead of, this one?

Authority – the information source

- Can you identify the author(s)? If not, the company/organisation/individuals behind the website should be considered the author.
- Consider their trustworthiness. What are the their educational credentials? Are they suitably and sufficiently qualified to write on the topic?
- While 'nutritionist' is not a protected term, a Board-Certified Veterinary Nutritionist is a registered trademark and is therefore reserved for use by suitably qualified veterinary specialists in animal nutrition. This is currently denoted by use of the post nominals DACVIM (Nutrition, Board Certified Veterinary Nutritionist) (Diplomat of the American College of Veterinary Internal Medicine (Nutrition)) and/or Dip ECVCN (EBVS European Specialist in Veterinary and Comparative Nutrition). Does the information source have a standing in the subject area and/or a relevant professional affiliation? Have they been cited elsewhere?
- Is the source a true expert in the field? The views of fake experts are often inconsistent with scientific evidence and disparaging against established researchers and true subject experts.
- Has the information been peer reviewed or critically evaluated?

Accuracy – the reliability, truthfulness and correctness of the content

- Where does the information come from?
- Is the content based on fact or personal experience/anecdote/opinion/propaganda?
- Is the information well reasoned and supported by an appropriate evidence base or existing literature? Are links to citations, other websites or information sources provided? If so, are these appropriate?
- Is there evidence that the content has been edited or peer reviewed?
- Can the information be verified by credible information sources?
- Are there spelling, grammar or typographical errors?

Continued

Table 3.2. Continued.

Purpose – the reason the information exists

- What is the purpose of the information? Is it to inform, educate, sell, entertain or persuade?
- Does it meet any personal, professional or societal needs?
- Does it have an economic value for the author or publisher?
- Are the intentions of the author(s) clear and transparent?
- Is the information objective and impartial or is there obvious or potential bias?
- Are there political, ideological, cultural, religious, institutional or personal biases?
- Does the information contain strong language or hyperbole?
- Are there any advertisements included in the source? If so, is there a relationship between the advertising and the content, or is it simply providing financial support?

Table 3.3. A look at the URL can help determine if it's a trustworthy website and reliable information source or not.

.org	An advocacy website, such as a not-for-profit organisation
.com	A business or commercial site
.edu	A site affiliated with an education institute
.gov	A government site
.net	A site from a network organisation or an internet service provider
.uk	indicative of the website's country of origin

Wherever possible, judgements about pet nutrition and other aspects of healthcare and welfare should be based on the best available, current, valid and relevant evidence. Alongside existing clinical expertise, informed risk management, excellent clinical reasoning and consideration of a pet's and/or caretaker's circumstances, preferences, beliefs and values, sound scientific evidence should guide clinical decision-making and help to educate and inform pet caretakers. However, not everyone values scientific evidence and not all evidence is equal (Murad *et al.*, 2016). The evidence pyramid (Fig. 3.6) was created to help visualise the quality and amount of available evidence. Inherent to this is the concept of a hierarchy, with improved validity and reliability, reduced risk of bias and statistical error, and greater effort and expertise associated with evidence at the top of the pyramid. It is useful to consider this when searching for evidence, appraising its quality and applying it, yet its accuracy cannot be guaranteed, and each design has its strengths and limitations (RCVS Knowledge, 2020). Furthermore, methodological limitations can affect the quality of evidence derived from any study design (Murad *et al.*, 2016). To further help in establishing the quality, trustworthiness and relevance of research findings and published evidence, critical appraisal tools are available, including those provided by the Centre for Evidence-based Veterinary Medicine (CEVM,

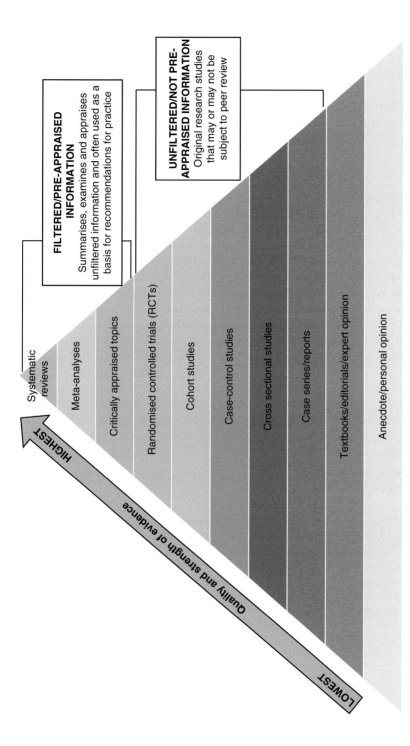

Fig. 3.6. An evidence pyramid illustrating the relative rigour, quality and reliability of information and evidence according to different study designs. Progression up the pyramid is associated with increasing quality, reliability and accuracy of evidence, in addition to reduced likelihood of statistical error or bias. Author's own figure.

2022), the Royal College of Veterinary Surgeons (RCVS Knowledge, 2022), the Critical Appraisal Skills Programme (CASP, 2022), the British Medical Journal (*BMJ*, 2022) and the Joanna Briggs Institute (JBI, 2020).

Dietary recommendations and policies should be guided by rigorous systematic reviews and meta-analyses, which are useful tools in summarising a large body of evidence and informing policy and guidelines (Tobias *et al.*, 2021; Zeraatkar *et al.*, 2021). However, these are scant in veterinary medicine and randomised controlled studies are more frequently used to inform dietary decision-making in relation to diet type and feeding management of a pet.

In summary

Nutrition is of critical importance to good health and wellbeing, to optimal growth and to the prevention and delayed progression of many disorders. Yet considerable confusion and misinformation exists regarding nutritional facts and dietary choice, with direct consequences on the health and wellbeing of veterinary patients, their caretakers and our relationships with clients. Not all pet caretakers trust the advice of the VHCT, instead relying on alternative sources of nutritional information with questionable accuracy, reliability and credibility. Educating about appropriate feeding protocols and diet choice helps to preserve the bond between pets and caretakers, therefore the VHCT should focus on optimum nutrition for every animal that presents to the practice. Wherever possible, decisions about pet diet selection and feeding management should be based on the highest available quality of scientific evidence. It is the responsibility of the VHCT to direct pet caretakers to appropriate, credible and accurate sources of information and to leverage the HAB when communicating with clients.

References

AAHA (2003) *The Path to High-quality Care: Practical tips for improving compliance.* American Animal Hospital Association, Lakewood, Colorado.

Adamski, M., Gibson, S., Leech, M. and Truby, H. (2018) Are doctors nutritionists? What is the role of doctors in providing nutrition advice? *Nutrition Bulletin,* 43, 147–152.

Alvarez, E.E., Schultz, K.K., Floerchinger, A.M. and Hull, J.L. (2022) Small animal general practitioners discuss nutrition infrequently despite assertion of indication, citing barriers. *Journal of the American Veterinary Medical Association,* 260 (13), 1704–1710.

Amiot, C., Bastian, B. and Martens, P. (2016) People and companion animals: it takes two to tango. *BioScience,* 66(7), 552–560.

Arai, T. (2014). The development of animal nutrition and metabolism and the challenges of our time. *Frontiers in Veterinary Science,* 1 (23), 1–3.

Becvarora, I., Prochazka, D., Chandler, M.L. and Meyer, H.J. (2016) Nutrition education in European veterinary schools: Are European veterinary graduates competent in nutrition? *Journal of Veterinary Medical Education,* 43(4), 349–358.

Bergler, R., Wechsung, S., Kienzle, E., Hoff, T. and Dobenecker, B. (2016) Nutrition consultation in small animal practice – a field for specialized veterinarians. *Tierarztl Prax Ausg K Kleintiere,* 44(1), 5–14.

BMJ (2022) How to read a paper. Available at: https://www.bmj.com/about-bmj/resources-readers/publications/how-read-paper (accessed 26 June 2022).

Boden, L. (2018) Pet owners turn to the internet for advice: will vets be there to provide an information prescription? *Veterinary Record,* 182, 599–600.

Bontempo, V. (2005) Nutrition and health of dogs and cats: Evolution of petfood. *Veterinary Research Communications,* 29, 45–50.

Boss, N., Ackerman, L., Donnelly, A.L., Rumple, S., Burns, K.M. *et al.* (2021) Client service considerations. In: Ackerman, L. (ed.) *Pet-Specific Care for the Veterinary Team.* Wiley, New Jersey, USA, pp. 291–292.

Bruckner, I. and Handl, S. (2020) Survey on the role of nutrition in first-opinion practices in Austria and Germany: An evaluation of knowledge, preferences and need for further education. *Journal of Animal Physiology and Animal Nutrition,* 105 (Suppl. 2), 89–94.

Brunetto, M.A., Gomes, M.O.S., Andre, M.R., Teshima, E., Gonçalves, K.N. *et al.* (2010) Effects of nutritional support on hospital outcome in dogs and cats. *Journal of Veterinary Emergency and Critical Care,* 20, 224–231.

Burns, K.M. (2014) Proper nutrition: Is the new emphasis a fad? *Veterinary Team Brief,* 2(3), 8–9.

BVA (2016) Pet obesity epidemic is top welfare concern for vets. Available at: https://www.bva.co.uk/news-and-blog/news-article/pet-obesity-epidemic-is-top-welfare-concern-for-vets/ (accessed 28 May 2022).

California State University (2010) Evaluating Information: Applying the CRAAP test. Available at: https://library.csuchico.edu/sites/default/files/craap-test.pdf (accessed 22 June 2022).

Carciofi, A.C. and Brunetto, A.M. (2009) Nutritional Support and hospital outcome: The importance of a positive caloric balance. Proceedings of the 34th WSAVA Veterinary Conference. Available at: http://www.vin.com/proceedings/Proceedings.plx?CID=WSAVA2009&Category=8054&PID=53618&O=Generic (accessed 26 June 2022).

Carlisle-Frank, P. and Frank, J.M. (2006) Owners, guardians, and owner guardians: Differing relationships with pets. *Anthrozoös,* 19, 225–242.

CASP (2022) CASP checklists. Available at: https://casp-uk.net/casp-tools-checklists/ (accessed 26 June 2022).

CEVM (2022) Centre for Evidence-based Veterinary Medicine – Our Resources. Available at: https://www.nottingham.ac.uk/cevm/resources/our-resources.aspx (accessed 23 June 2022).

Chan, D.L., Freeman, L.M., Labato, M.A. and Rush, J.E. (2002) Retrospective evaluation of partial parenteral nutrition in dogs and cats. *Journal of Veterinary Internal Medicine,* 16(4), 440–445.

Chandler, M. (2018) Busting pet nutrition myths. *In Focus.* Available at: https://www.veterinary-practice.com/article/busting-pet-nutrition-myths (accessed 9 September 2022).

Cohen, S.P. (2002) Can pets function as family members? *Western Journal of Nursing Research,* 24, 621–638.

Connolly, K.M., Heinze, C.R. and Freeman, L.M. (2014) Feeding practices of dog breeders in the United States and Canada. *Journal of the American Veterinary Medical Association*, 245(6), 669–676.

Conway, D.M.P. and Saker, K.E. (2018) Consumer Attitude Toward the Environmental Sustainability of Grain-Free Pet Foods. *Frontiers in Veterinary Science*, 5, 1–8.

Empert-Gallegos, A., Poole, S. and Yam, P. (2020) Raw insights into dog owner perspectives on risks, benefits, and nutritional value of raw diets compared to cooked diets. *Peer J*, 8: e10383.

Epley, N., Waytz, A. and Cacioppo, J.T. (2007) On seeing human: A three-factor theory of anthropomorphism. *Psychological Review*, 114, 864.

Evason, M., Peace, M., Munguia, G. and Stull, J. (2020) Clients' knowledge, attitudes, and practices related to pet nutrition and exercise at a teaching hospital. *The Canadian Veterinary Journal*, 61(5), 512–516.

FEDIAF (2022a) Health benefits. Available at: https://europeanpetfood.org/pets-in-society/health-benefits/ (accessed 25 June 2022).

FEDIAF (2022b) Pet food industry trends. Available at: https://fediaf.org/prepared-pet-foods/pet-food-trends.html (accessed 25 June 2022).

Fifield, S.J. and Forsyth, D.K. (1999) A pet for the children: Factors related to family pet ownership. *Anthrozoös*, 12(1), 24–32.

Flocke, A., Thiemeyera, H. and Kiefer-Hecker, B. (2013) Dog and cat nutrition practices of owners visiting veterinary clinics. In: European Society of Veterinary and Comparative Nutrition. (ed.) *Proceedings of the 17th Congress of the ESVCN*, Ghent, Belgium, pp. 19–21.

Friedmann, E. and Son, H. (2009) The human–companion animal bond: How humans benefit. *Veterinary Clinics of North America: Small Animal Practice*, 39(2), 293–326.

Gadomski, A.M., Scribani, M.B., Krupa, N. and Jenkins, P. (2017) Pet dogs and child physical activity: the role of child–dog attachment. *Pediatric Obesity*, 12(5), e37–40.

Gee, N.R., Fine, A.H., and McCardle, P. (2017). *How Animals Help Students Learn: Research and Practice for Educators and Mental-Health Professionals,* 1st edn. Routledge, New York, USA.

Gee, N.R. and Mueller, M,K. (2019) A systematic review of research on pet ownership and animal interactions among older adults. *Anthrozoös*, 32(2), 183–207.

HABRI (2022) What is the human-animal bond? Available at: https://habri.org/about/ (accessed 17 June 2022).

Hamburg, M. E., Finkenauer, C. and Schuengel, C. (2014) Food for love: the role of food offering in empathic emotion regulation. *Frontiers in Psychology*, 5, 32.

Harris, J. P., Parnell, N. K., Griffith, E. H. and Saker, K.E. (2017) Retrospective evaluation of the impact of early enteral nutrition on clinical outcomes in dogs with pancreatitis: 34 cases (2010–2013). *Journal of Veterinary Emergency and Critical Care*, 27, 425–433.

Herzog, H.A. (2014) Biology, culture, and the origins of pet-keeping. *Animal Behavior and Cognition,* 1(3), 296–308.

Holbrook, M.B. (1996) Reflections of Rocky. *Society and Animals,* 4 (20), 147–168.

JBI (2020) Critical Appraisal Tools. Available at: https://jbi.global/critical-appraisal-tools (accessed 23 June 2022).

Johnson, J. (2022) The importance of the human-animal bond for the veterinary profession. Available at: https://habri.org/hab-lectures?view-session=the-importance-of-the-human-animal-bond-for-the-veterinary-profession (accessed 19 June 2022).

Kathrani, A. (2016) Nutritional support in the intensive care unit. *In Practice*, 38, 18–24.

Kealy, R.D., Lawler, D.F., Ballam, J.M., Mantz, S.L., Biery, D.N. *et al.* (2002) Effects of diet restriction on life span and age-related changes in dogs. *Journal of the American Veterinary Medical Association,* 220(9), 1315–1320.

Kienzle, E., Bergler, R. and Mandernach, A. (1998) A comparison of the feeding behavior and the human-animal relationship in owners of normal and obese dogs. *Journal of Nutrition*, 128(12 Suppl.), 2779S –2782S.

Kipperman, B.S. and German, A.J. (2018) The responsibility of veterinarians to address companion animal obesity. *Animals (Basel)*, 8(9), 143.

Kogan, L. and Oxley, J.A. (2020) Nurses' views of pet owners: Online pet health information. *The Veterinary Nurse*, 11(8), 379–383.

Kogan, L.R., Goldwaser, G., Stewart, S.M. and Schoenfeld-Tacher, R. (2008) Sources and frequency of use of pet health information and level of confidence in information accuracy, as reported by owners visiting small animal veterinary practices. *Journal of the American Veterinary Medical Association*, 232(10), 1536–1542.

Kogan, L.R., Schoenfeld-Tacher, R., Simon, A. and Viera, A.R. (2010) The internet and pet health information: Perceptions and behaviors of pet owners and veterinarians. *The Internet Journal of Veterinary Medicine,* 8(1).

Kogan, L.R., Schoenfeld-Tacher, R. and Viera, A.R. (2012) The internet and health information: differences in pet owners based on age, gender, and education. *Journal of the Medical Library Association,* 100(3), 197– 204.

Kogan, L.R., Schoenfeld-Tacher, R., Gould, L., Hellyer, P.W. and Dowers, K. (2014) Information prescriptions: A tool for veterinary practices. *Open Veterinary Journal,* 4(2), 90–95.

Kogan, L., Oxley, J.A., Hellyer, P., Schoenfeld, R. and Rishniw, M. (2018) UK pet owners' use of the internet for online pet health information. *Veterinary Record*, 182(21), 601.

Kogan, L., Hazel, S. and Oxley, J. (2019) A pilot study of Australian pet owners who engage in social media and their use, experience and views of online pet health information. *Australian Veterinary Journal*, 97, 433–439.

Kogan, L.R., Little, S. and Oxley, J. (2021) Dog and cat owners' use of online Facebook groups for pet health information. *Health Information and Libraries Journal*, 38, 203–223.

Kuhl, C.A., Lea, R.G., Quarmby, C. and Dean, R. (2022) Scoping review to assess online information available to new dog owners. *Veterinary Record,* 190 (10), e1487.

Lai, N., Khosa, D.K., Jones-Bitton, A. and Dewey, C.E. (2021) Pet owners' online information searches and the perceived effects on interactions and relationships with their veterinarians. *The Veterinary Evidence,* 6(1), 1–15.

Lancendorfer, K.M., Atkin, J.L. and Reece, B.B. (2008) Animals in advertising: Love dogs? Love the ad! *Journal of Business Research,* 61(5), 384–391.

Larsen, J.A. and Villaverde, C. (2016) Scope of the problem and perception by owners and veterinarians. *Veterinary Clinics of North America: Small Animal Practice,* 46(5), 761–772.

Liu, D.T., Brown, D.C. and Silverstein, D.C. (2012) Early nutritional support is associated with decreased length of hospitalization in dogs with septic peritonitis: a retrospective study of 45 cases (2000–2009). *Journal of Veterinary Emergency and Critical Care,* 22, 453–459

Lue, T.W., Pantenburg, D.P. and Crawford, P.M. (2008). Impact of the owner–pet and client–veterinarian bond on the care that pets receive. *Journal of the American Veterinary Medical Association*, 232(4), 531–540.

Lumbis, R. and de Scally, M. (2020) Knowledge, attitudes and application of nutrition assessments by the veterinary health care team in small animal practice. *Journal of Small Animal Practice,* 61, 494–503.

Mansfield, C. and Beths, T. (2015) Management of acute pancreatitis in dogs: A critical appraisal with focus on feeding and analgesia. *Journal of Small Animal Practice,* 56, 27–39.

McCullough, A., Jenkins, M., Ruehrdanz, A., Gilmer, M.J., Olson, J. *et al.* (2018) Physiological and behavioral effects of animal-assisted interventions for therapy dogs in pediatric oncology settings. *Applied Animal Behaviour Science,* 200, 86–95.

Michel, K.E., Willoughby, K.N., Abood, S.K., Fascetti, A.J., Fleeman, L.M. *et al.* (2008) Attitudes of pet owners toward pet foods and feeding management of cats and dogs. *Journal of the American Veterinary Medical Association,* 233(11), 1699–1703.

Mohr, A.J., Leisewitz, A.L., Jacobson, L.S., Steiner, J.M., Ruaux, C.G. *et al.* (2003) Effect of early enteral nutrition on intestinal permeability, intestinal protein loss, and outcome in dogs with severe parvoviral enteritis. *Journal of Veterinary Internal Medicine,* 17, 791–798.

Morgan, S.K., Willis, S. and Shepherd, M.L. (2017) Survey of owner motivations and veterinary input of owners feeding diets containing raw animal products. *Peer J,* 5, e3031.

Murad, M.H., Asi, N., Alsawas, M. and Alahdab, F. (2016) New evidence pyramid. *British Medical Journal Evidence-Based Medicine,* 21(4), 125–127.

Murphy, S.A. (2006) Consumer health information for pet owners. *Journal of the Medical Library Association,* 94, 151–158.

Oxley, J.A., Eastwood, B. and Kogan, L.R. (2017) Pet owners and the internet. *Companion Animal,* 22(6), 358–358.

PDSA (2021) 2021 PDSA Animal Wellbeing (PAW) Report: Diet and obesity. Available at: https://www.pdsa.org.uk/what-we-do/pdsa-animal-wellbeing-report/paw-report-2021/diet-and-obesity (accessed 19 May 2022).

Pet Food Industry (2020) New study reveals COVID-19 pandemic fueling pet obesity. Available at: https://www.petfoodindustry.com/articles/9877-new-study-reveals-covid-19-pandemic-fueling-pet-obesity (accessed 26 June 2022).

PFMA (2022) *2022 Annual Report.* Available at https://pfma-reports.co.uk/ (accessed 22 December 2022)

Poresky, R.H. (1990) The young children's empathy measure: Reliability, validity and effects of companion animal bonding. *Psychological Reports,* 66(3), 931–936.

RCVS Knowledge (2020) EBVM Toolkit. Available at: https://knowledge.rcvs.org.uk/evidence-based-veterinary-medicine/ebvm-toolkit/ (accessed 23 July 2022).

RCVS Knowledge (2022) EBVM Toolkit 3 – Introduction to 'levels of evidence' and study design. Available at: https://knowledge.rcvs.org.uk/document-library/ebvm-toolkit-3-introduction-to-levels-of-evidence-and-study/ (accessed 23 July 2022).

Remillard, R.L., Darden, D.E., Michel, K.E., Marks, S.L. and Buffington, C.A. *et al.* (2001) An investigation of the relationship between caloric intake and outcome in hospitalised dogs. *Veterinary Therapeutics,* 2, 301–310

Sallander, M. and Jaktlund, A. (2012/2013) Use of veterinary diets for dogs and cats hospitalized at a veterinary university clinic in Sweden. *The Veterinary Nurse,* 3, 638–644.

Sandøe, P., Corr, S. and Palmer, C. (2014) Fat companions: understanding the welfare effects of obesity in cats and dogs. In: Appleby, M.C., Weary, D.M. and Sandøe, P. (eds.) *Dilemmas in Animal Welfare.* CABI, Oxfordshire, UK.

Sapowicz, S.A., Linder, D.E. and Freeman, L.M. (2016) Body condition scores and evaluation of feeding habits of dogs and cats at a low cost veterinary clinic and a general practice. *Scientific World Journal,* 2016, 1901679.

Schleicher, M., Cash, S.B. and Freeman, L.M. (2019) Determinants of pet food purchasing decisions. *The Canadian Veterinary Journal*, 60, 644–650.

Simonsen, J.E., Fasenko, G.M. and Lillywhite, J.M. (2014) The Value-Added Dog Food Market: Do Dog Owners Prefer Natural or Organic Dog Foods? *Journal of Agricultural Science*, 6(6), 86–97.

Solhjoo, N., Naghshineh, N. and Fahimnia, F. (2017) The internet and pet health: Case study of online health information seeking behaviour of pet owners. *Journal of Information Systems and Services,* 6(1,2), 1–16.

Solhjoo, N., Naghshineh, N., Fahimnia, F. and Ameri-Naeini, A.R. (2018) Interventions to assist pet owners in online health information seeking behaviour: a qualitative content analysis literature review and proposed model. *Health Information and Libraries Journal*, 35(4), 265–284.

Statista (2022) Number of internet and social media users worldwide as of July 2022. Available at: https://www.statista.com/statistics/617136/digital-population-worldwide/ (accessed 21 December 2022)

Tobias, D.K., Wittenbecher, C. and Hu, F.B. (2021) Grading nutrition evidence: where to go from here? *American Journal of Clinical Nutrition*, 113(6), 1385–1387.

Vidović, V.V., Štetić, V.V. and Bratko, D. (1999) Pet ownership, type of pet and socio-emotional development of school children, *Anthrozoös*, 12(4), 211–217.

Wainwright, J., Millar, K.M. and White, G.A. (2022) Owners' views of canine nutrition, weight status and wellbeing and their implications for the veterinary consultation. *Journal of Small Animal Practice*, 63, 381–388.

Wanser, S.H., Vitale, K.R., Thielke, L.E., Brubaker, L. and Udell, M.A. (2019) Spotlight on the psychological basis of childhood pet attachment and its implications. *Psychology Research and Behavior Management*, 12, 469–479.

Ward, E., German, A.J. and Churchill, J.A. (2019) The global pet obesity initiative position statement. Available at: https://static1.squarespace.com/static/597c-71d3e58c621d06830e3f/t/5da311c5519bf62664dac512/1570968005938/Global+pet+obesity+initiative+position+statement.pdf (accessed 28 May 2022)

Wedderburn, P. (2022) 'Fur babies' and the future of pet care at innovation summit. *Veterinary Times,* 52(8), 22.

Wensley, S.P. (2008) Animal welfare and the human-animal bond: considerations for veterinary faculty, students, and practitioners. *Journal of Veterinary Medical Education,* 35(4), 532–539.

Westgarth, C., Heron, J., Ness, A.R., Bundred, P., Gaskell, R.M., Coyne, K.P., German A.J., McCune S. and Dawson, S. (2010) Family pet ownership during childhood: Findings from a UK birth cohort and implications for public health research. *International Journal of Environmental Research and Public Health*, 7, 3704–3729.

WSAVA (2013a) The savvy dog owner's guide: Nutrition on the internet. Available at: https://wsava.org/wp-content/uploads/2020/01/The-Savvy-Dog-Owner-s-Guide-to-Nutrition-on-the-Internet.pdf (accessed 20 June 2022).

WSAVA (2013b) The savvy cat owner's guide: Nutrition on the internet. Available at: https://wsava.org/wp-content/uploads/2020/01/The-Savvy-Cat-Owner-s-Guide-to-Nutrition-on-the-Internet.pdf (accessed 20 June 2022).

Yam, P.S., Naughton, G., Butowski, C.F. and Root, A.L. (2017) Inaccurate assessment of canine body condition score, bodyweight, and pet food labels: a potential cause of inaccurate feeding. *Veterinary Sciences*, 4(2), 30.

Zeraatkar, D., Bhasin, A., Morassut, R.E., Churchill, I., Gupta, A. *et al.* (2021) Characteristics and quality of systematic reviews and meta-analyses of observational nutritional epidemiology: a cross-sectional study. *American Journal of Clinical Nutrition*, 113(6), 1578–1592.

Nutrition as the fifth vital sign

4

Rachel Lumbis

Abstract

Nutrition is one of the most important considerations in the maintenance of health, and early intervention can play a critical role in ensuring successful patient outcome and management of disease (Kealy *et al.*, 2002; Mohr *et al.*, 2003; Liu *et al.*, 2012). In veterinary patients, this is reflected by the recognition of nutritional assessment as the fifth vital assessment following the evaluation of temperature, pulse, respiration and pain (Freeman *et al.*, 2011). However, despite freely available and accessible nutritional assessment guidelines, tools and resources, knowledge and/or the motivation to use these appears deficient within veterinary practice and it is an often-overlooked aspect of veterinary care. Every pet should undergo a nutritional assessment at every visit to determine an appropriate quantity and type of food, and the most effective feeding method. This chapter will outline the World Small Animal Veterinary Association (WSAVA) Nutritional Assessment Guidelines and resources, and suggest ways to effectively incorporate nutritional awareness, assessment and support into clinical practice as a crucial component of patient care.

Nutritional assessment

As with any medical intervention, there are always risks of complications and this is no different with nutritional interventions. Minimising such risks depends on regular nutritional assessment (NA), prompt identification of patients in need of nutritional support and determination of the optimal diet, daily food allowance, feeding route and method. Following the evaluation of temperature, pulse, respiration and pain, NA is the fifth vital assessment and identifies malnourished patients requiring immediate nutritional support, as well as those at risk of developing malnutrition (Freeman *et al.*, 2011). Regardless of age, life stage and condition, an NA should be conducted on every pet that is presented at the veterinary practice as part of routine history taking and physical examination.

© Rachel Lumbis and Tierney Kinnison 2023. *An Interprofessional Approach to Veterinary Nutrition* (R. Lumbis and T. Kinnison)
DOI: 10.1079/9781800621107.0004

To help the veterinary healthcare team (VHCT) and pet caretakers in ensuring that small animals receive optimal nutrition, tailored to their needs, the WSAVA Global Nutrition Committee launched its Nutritional Assessment Guidelines in 2011 (Freeman *et al.*, 2011). These are based on the American Animal Hospital Association (AAHA) Nutritional Assessment Guidelines (Baldwin *et al.*, 2010) and have since been published worldwide and translated into 12 different languages. For the VHCT, these guidelines provide a framework to assist in making an NA, and in providing specific nutritional recommendations, for small animal patients at every visit (Fig. 4.1).

The first stage involves making an initial, systematic 'screening' evaluation of the animal, as well as identification of the diet being fed and a review of feeding management and environmental factors. It is also important to consider any human-related factors associated with a dog's or cat's nutrition (Cline *et al.*, 2021). A comprehensive nutrition history, containing accurate and honest information about the pet's normal feeding habits and preferences at home, must be obtained from the caretaker. A veterinarian may not always be the most appropriate member of the VHCT to acquire this; some caretakers may prefer to have a discussion with, and ask questions of, a non-veterinarian

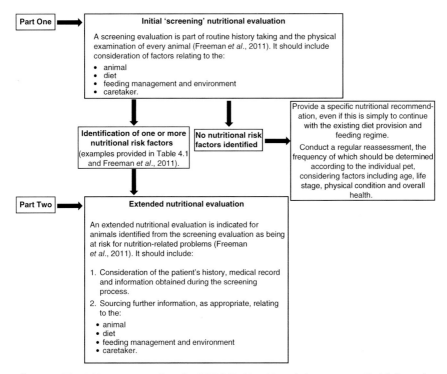

Fig. 4.1. The NA process using the WSAVA Nutritional Assessment Guidelines for Dogs and Cats. Author's own figure.

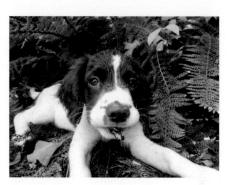

Fig. 4.2. When taking a nutritional history, it is essential to question caretakers about their pet's consumption of conventional food and supplements, as well as items not intended, or suitable, for consumption. The presentation of a puppy or kitten for a health check is an ideal opportunity to raise the topic and advise caretakers about optimal diet and feeding choices, helping to normalise nutrition conversations throughout the pet's life. Photograph: author.

(AAHA, 2009). When questioning clients about an animal's nutritional intake, it is important to consider conventional food and supplements that the care-taker intends for their pet's consumption, as well as unconventional 'food', not intended for consumption (Fig. 4.2).

A screening evaluation may indicate that a pet is in good health and physical condition, is being housed in appropriate environmental conditions and is being fed a suitable and adequate diet with optimal feeding management. In this situation, the recommendation and plan may simply be to continue with the current regime and to regularly reassess this. The exact frequency should be based on the species, breed, age/life stage, health status and environment of each individual pet. Life stage may influence the approach taken to conducting an NA of a dog or cat, with specific considerations outlined for each stage outlined by AAHA (2021a) and AAHA (2021b). Healthy pregnant, lactating, senior, and growing animals require more frequent monitoring (Freeman *et al.*, 2011).

The identification, or suspected presence, of any nutrition-related risk factors (Table 4.1), including previous or ongoing medical conditions or disease, prompts a more in-depth 'extended' evaluation of each of these factors, a framework for which is published online (AAHA, 2010). Regardless of whether nutritional risk factors are present, it is important to make a specific dietary recommendation and nutritional plan, while also considering the preferences of the pet and care-taker. A nutritional plan should prevent (or correct) overt nutritional deficien-cies and imbalances. Using the APIE (Assessment, Planning, Implementing and Evaluating) approach, first outlined by Yura and Walsh (1967) in relation to care planning, offers a systematic and recurrent approach to nutritional planning.

Non-hospitalised animals will require regular reassessment to ensure optimisation of nutritional intake, with appropriate adjustments made where

Table 4.1. Factors to consider when making an initial, systematic 'screening' evaluation, as outlined in the WSAVA Nutritional Assessment Guidelines, and examples of associated nutritional risk factors.

	Animal-specific factors	Diet-specific factors	Feeding management and environmental factors	Human-related factors
Initial 'screening' evaluation	• Species and breed • Age • Physiological status • Health status and presence of disease • Body weight • Body condition score (BCS) • Muscle condition score (MCS) • Exercise and activity level	• Safety, appropriateness and nutritional adequacy of the diet • Animal preference • Caretaker preference	• Frequency, timing, location and method of feeding • Space and suitability of the pet's surroundings	Consideration of the caretaker's: • beliefs • culture • financial situation • relationship and bond with their pet
Examples of nutritional risk factors	• BCS of less than 4/9 or over 5/9 • Any degree of muscle wastage • Unexplained weight change, particularly any unintentional weight loss of 10% or more body weight • Altered feeding behaviour or intake • Altered gastrointestinal function (e.g. vomiting, diarrhoea, flatulence, constipation) • Evidence of medical conditions and disease (existing or current) • Receiving medications	• Concerns over safety or appropriateness of the diet being fed • Snacks, treats, table food constituting over 10% of daily caloric intake • The feeding of an unconventional diet (e.g. plant-based, raw meat-based or home prepared-cooked) • Provision of dietary supplements • Evidence of nutrient imbalances and spoilage or contamination of the diet	• Inadequate or inappropriate housing and husbandry • Over- or underfeeding • Excessive use of treats • Competitive eating • Lack of appropriate environmental stimulation and enrichment • Identification of environmental stressors • Insufficient daily activity or exercise level	Identification of factors that may be discordant to the provision of an appropriate, safe and optimal diet for the pet

necessary to achieve and maintain optimal body condition (Freeman *et al.*, 2011). Specific nutritional management is indicated as part of the treatment of a variety of chronic conditions affecting both humans and pets in the UK, including obesity, cancer, heart disease and diabetes. It is therefore essential to encourage the active involvement of all caretakers in the NA of their pet(s) at home. Providing instruction on how to accurately assess body and muscle condition, alongside the consideration of other important factors, is crucial to early detection of disease in all life-stages, with Freeman *et al.* (2011) recommending regular assessment of:

- food intake and appetite
- body condition score and body weight
- gastrointestinal signs (e.g. faecal consistency and volume; any vomiting)
- overall appearance and activity.

The feeding plan formulated for a hospitalised animal must include the most appropriate method and route of delivery, alongside the patient's nutritional and energy requirements and feeding goals. It should be completed in consultation with the animal's caretaker, and any underlying disease process, clinical signs and the anticipated duration of nutritional support should be determined and factored into the plan. This information must be documented on patient records and as part of a comprehensive nursing care plan, with prescribed feeding orders clearly communicated to all those involved in patient care and treatment. It should be reviewed daily, together with the evaluation of:

- specific food orders, including diet, route, amount and frequency
- route of intake and whether this is still optimal
- quantification of nutrient intake (via all routes)
- fluid balance
- relevant clinical signs or diagnostic tests.

Daily monitoring and evaluation of patient dietary requirements and nutrition support is essential to determine the progression of a patient's health and nutritional status and to examine whether goals and expected outcomes are being met. It also enables the rapid identification of any complications and deterioration in condition.

Establishing good client rapport and making use of appropriate communication is crucial to achieving desired outcomes (Cornell and Kopcha, 2007; Michel, 2009; Creevy *et al.*, 2019; Quimby *et al.*, 2021). During each consultation, or on a pet's discharge from the hospital, a clearly documented, specific dietary recommendation and nutritional plan should be formulated in consultation with the caretaker. This should be based on shared knowledge and common goals, ideas, beliefs and expectations, and include the recommended diet, feeding method, caloric intake, frequency of feeding and the schedule for rechecks and reassessment. It is important to provide caretakers with a hard copy of this information and clear explanation of the reasons for the recommended feeding plan, alongside an opportunity to ask questions (Cline *et al.*, 2021).

Compliance with nutritional recommendations can be further maximised through the following.

- **Good teamwork**, with appropriate delegation and the utilisation of all members of the VHCT to provide feeding advice and caretaker support in executing nutritional recommendations and reinforcing a nutritional plan (Freeman *et al.*, 2011; Cline *et al.*, 2021). Further information can be found in subsequent chapters, with patient-based examples in Chapters 8 and 10.
- **Encouraging caretakers to take an active role** in the decision-making process and planning of their pet's dietary management and other aspects of veterinary healthcare and treatment (concordance) (Johnson and Linder, 2013).
- **Ensuring parity between the viewpoints of the VHCT and pet caretaker**, ensuring that the nutritional recommendation is tailored to the client's perceptions and beliefs (Kamleh *et al.*, 2020).
- Understanding the factors affecting whether a client will comply with the specified dietary recommendations and **identifying any issues that may limit client adherence** (Michel, 2009; Freeman *et al.*, 2011).
- **Planning for maintained contact with caretakers after their pet's visit** to improve accountability, resolve any problems and address any queries or concerns (Wareham *et al.*, 2019).
- **Maintaining regular communication with caretakers as a dialogue**, rather than a lecture, with continued demonstration of reflective listening and empathy (Johnson and Linder, 2013; Cline *et al.*, 2021).

Scheduling follow-up appointments as part of a thorough nutritional assessment and record of the nutritional recommendation in the pet's medical records will help to establish nutrition as a routine part of patient care. It will also:

- prompt a review of the nutritional recommendation and enable any necessary adjustments to be made
- allow the caretaker to ask questions
- enable trends to be monitored
- reinforce the desire of the VHCT to form a partnership with the caretaker to achieve the best for their pet.

The Global Nutrition Toolkit

Following on from the launch of the WSAVA's Global Nutrition Guidelines in 2011, a suite of non-branded support materials and practical aids has been developed by the WSAVA Global Nutrition Committee as part of the Global Nutrition Toolkit (WSAVA, 2021). These are freely available to access and download from the WSAVA website (https://wsava.org/global-guidelines/global-nutrition-guidelines/).

Tools including a dietary history form, NA checklist and calorie chart for healthy dogs and cats, help the VHCT to address nutrition at every patient visit and assist in making NA and recommendations more efficient. Guidance for the nutritional support of clinically affected patients is also provided through feeding guides, feeding instructions and a monitoring chart for hospitalised dogs and cats, together with videos illustrating placement of common feeding tubes. The availability of body and muscle condition score charts and videos facilitates consistency in use across the VHCT and pet caretakers. Guidance for successful implementation, including communication tips, helps to further advance the central role of the VHCT as the expert source of nutrition information.

Several non-branded educational materials have also been designed specifically for pet caretakers. These assist in making appropriate pet diet-related decisions, help to clarify common dietary myths and misconceptions and educate about different diets and pet food ingredients. They also help to promote caretaker provision of a full and accurate nutrition history.

Barriers to implementation

The WSAVA guidelines are the accepted standard of NA and should form part of the minimum standard of care. While awareness of the concept is apparent, an NA is often neglected and is seldom completed in full, or discussed with caretakers, at every veterinary visit (German and Morgan, 2008; Rolph et al., 2014; Bergler et al., 2016; Vandendriessche et al., 2017; Santarossa et al., 2018; Bruckner and Handl, 2020; Lumbis and de Scally, 2020; Blees et al., 2021; Alvarez et al., 2022). Furthermore, there is limited, or no, consideration of pets' dietary intake and formal dietary records are not being kept for all patients, whether healthy or sick (Rolph et al., 2014; Lumbis and de Scally, 2020). The reasons for this disconnect are numerous and include:

- an under-representation of nutrition education at many veterinary schools with limited nutrition-related curriculum content (Becvarova et al., 2016)
- perceived suboptimal skills, incompetence and a lack of knowledge and understanding of basic nutrition principles and interventions to counsel clients effectively (Sallander and Jaktlund, 2012/2013; Bergler et al., 2016; Siebert et al., 2016; Bruckner and Handl, 2020)
- concerns about time constraints with too tight a schedule or short appointment times and perceived insufficient time for an NA and/or discussion about diet (German and Morgan 2008; Alvarez et al., 2022)
- a lack of confidence to discuss diet and nutrition with pet caretakers (Chandler and Takashima, 2014; Bergler et al., 2016; Lumbis and de Scally, 2020) and difficulty keeping up with products (Alvarez et al., 2022) (communicating effectively with caretakers about dietary management of companion animals can be difficult, particularly when the goal is to persuade a pet caretaker to alter feeding practices) (Michel, 2009)

- perception by the practice team that NA is of limited importance, unless directly relevant to a patient's presenting complaint (Bruckner and Handl, 2020)
- impact of the coronavirus pandemic, with virtual veterinary appointments on the rise, meaning declining pet caretaker visits to veterinary practices and fewer NAs being performed in person
- clients' perceptions and concerns about the effectiveness of veterinary nutritional recommendations (Kamleh *et al.*, 2020)
- clients' lack of awareness and acceptance of the importance of optimal pet nutrition and/or belief that it is purely an opportunity to generate revenue
- caretakers question the motivations behind nutritional recommendations, particularly when they involve a commercial pet food (Cline *et al.*, 2021) and may be resistant to changing brand (Alvarez *et al.*, 2022).

Consistent implementation of NA in the hospital setting is also lacking. WSAVA guidelines suggest that, unless contraindicated, all hospitalised animals should have their resting energy requirements (RER) calculated, an appropriate diet prescribed, and feeding instructions clearly detailed on their hospital chart. Actual amount eaten must also be recorded and, if insufficient, an assisted feeding plan or nutritional intervention must be implemented (Freeman *et al.*, 2011). Despite this, the use of freely available feeding guides, monitoring charts, calorie calculation charts and other NA tools is inconsistent (Lumbis and de Scally, 2020) and malnutrition of hospitalised patients in small animal veterinary hospitals is well documented (Remillard *et al.*, 2001; Chandler and Gunn-Moore, 2004; Molina *et al.*, 2018). Nutritional intervention is frequently delayed, even in patients admitted with a history of altered food intake (Chandler and Gunn-Moore, 2004; Villaverde and Larsen, 2015) and development of nutrition-related diseases often precedes the provision of dietary recommendations (Rolph *et al.*, 2014; MacMartin *et al.*, 2015; Bergler *et al.*, 2016; Siebert *et al.*, 2016). Complete and accurate records of nutrition history and recommendations are essential for continuity of patient care and help to ensure the critical tracking and evaluation of the impact of nutrition on ongoing changes in health and wellbeing. The formulation of a feeding plan, alone, fails to guarantee delivery of the required caloric and dietary intake (Remillard *et al.*, 2001).

Incorporating nutritional awareness, assessment and support into clinical practice

Irregularity in the completion of a full NA, as described by the WSAVA guidelines, can cause nutritional risk factors to go unnoticed, with significant consequences for patient care (Bergler *et al.*, 2016; Vandendriessche *et al.*, 2017) and a reactive, instead of a proactive, attitude towards nutrition (Bergler *et al.*, 2016; Blees *et al.*, 2021). A consistent and detailed approach, involving all members of the VHCT, is fundamental to effective NA and the provision of dietary recommendations and protocols. By working together and utilising the many tools available to make nutritional conservation and assessment easier and faster, many of the acknowledged challenges in implementation can be overcome.

Clients who understand that preventive care preserves and lengthens their relationship with their pets are more likely to use veterinary services regularly, so team members should focus on proper nutrition for every patient that presents to their practice. As acknowledged by the alleged Hippocratic phrase 'let food be thy medicine and medicine be thy food' (Cardenas, 2013), good nutrition is *not* a fad – it is good business and good medicine. An understanding of basic nutritional principles and the application of nutrition in optimising the health and wellbeing of both fit and clinically affected companion animals is therefore essential for all members of the VHCT.

Making a dietary assessment

A continued expansion of the pet food market may prohibit a thorough knowledge of every available diet. Yet, all veterinary and veterinary nursing practitioners should be able to provide, at minimum, advice regarding fundamental and life-stage-appropriate nutritional requirements and be sufficiently skilled to conduct a basic assessment of the diet being fed.

Finding out exactly what, when and how much a pet caretaker is feeding is essential to ensure that the diet is appropriate for the intended species, life stage and health status of the animal and can meet its nutritional requirements. It is further crucial for the identification of potential problems, including:

- unbalanced or incomplete diets
- poor quality or unsafe diets that contain contaminants or pathogens
- inappropriate snacks, treats and supplements (including food being given to enable the administration of medication)
- inappropriate amount of food being offered.

Obtaining an accurate and complete nutrition history requires caretakers to be honest and sufficiently informed and detailed about the type and amount of food being offered to their pet. Emailing a nutrition screening survey or having one available at reception for pet caretakers to complete prior to elective appointments, together with an explanation of why this information is being requested, is one way to help achieve this. Completion at home can help increase the accuracy of information provided as well as reducing any perceived pressure or judgement felt by caretakers (Churchill and Ward, 2016).

When time is short:

- Utilise the entire VHCT, especially in the nutritional assessment process and in the communication of, and follow-up to, nutrition recommendations. They are a valuable resource in the education and support of pet caretakers.

- Obtain a nutrition history prior to the pet's arrival and encourage the caretaker to bring in photos of the diet(s) they are feeding and any supplements.
- Talk about nutrition while completing a physical examination.
- Use freely available resources (highlighted here and in Chapter 3) to assist with performing an NA and educating clients, and when communicating a nutritional recommendation.

Factors contributing to the successful implementation of nutrition assessment and support

Reported contributory factors to the successful implementation of NA and provision of dietary recommendations and protocols include:

- creating awareness among the VHCT and pet caretakers about the importance of NA, planning and intervention
- making a team commitment to acknowledge nutrition as the fifth vital assessment and following the WSAVA Nutritional Assessment Guidelines
- collaborating to develop a customised written protocol to ensure every patient receives an NA and specific dietary recommendation at every visit
- ensuring appropriate team training so that all staff, from reception and administration through to veterinary nurses/technicians and veterinarians, are sufficiently knowledgeable, competent and confident to follow practice protocols
- promoting client education and effective communication about nutrition as a key responsibility for all members of the VHCT (further information about broaching the subject of nutrition can be found in Chapter 7)
- effectively communicating prescribed feeding orders to all those involved in patient care and treatment
- ensuring accurate record-keeping, including the completion of a separate nutrition monitoring chart
- identifying, training, and utilising a nutrition 'champion' to help promote the inclusion of nutrition as a standard component of patient care and to reinforce good nutritional practice throughout the veterinary clinic (Creevy *et al.*, 2019)
- incorporating NA as a (mandatory) field in patient records to increase the frequency of performed NAs (Blees *et al.*, 2021).

Such factors highlight the importance of interprofessional collaboration between personnel, patient planning and the provision of explicit instruction. As acknowledged by the AAHA (2009), the provision of high-quality patient care can be achieved when every member of the pet's healthcare team, including the caretaker, shares a common understanding and agreement about all aspects of the recommended care.

In summary

NA is an important, yet often overlooked, aspect of veterinary care that should be embraced as a valuable diagnostic tool. Incorporating NA into patient care is critical to the optimisation of animal health and enhancement of pets' quality of life. It also strengthens relationships with clients, helping to facilitate a partnership and build trust between the pet caretaker and the VHCT, resulting in better care and healthier pets. Once dietary intervention is deemed necessary, collaboration is essential to determine the most appropriate method and route of delivery, the patient's nutrient and energy requirements, and feeding goals, and to ensure effective monitoring. Appropriate delegation and utilisation of all members of the VHCT is crucial to providing consistency in and continuity of patient care, optimal dietary advice and pet caretaker support in executing nutritional recommendations.

References

AAHA (American Animal Hospital Association) (2009) *Six Steps to Higher-quality Patient care*. AAHA Press, Lakewood, Colorado.

AAHA (American Animal Hospital Association) (2010) Extended nutrition evaluations. Available at: https://www.aaha.org/globalassets/02-guidelines/nutritional-assessment/nutritionevaluationform.pdf (accessed 29 January 2022).

AAHA (American Animal Hospital Association) (2021a) Nutrition and weight management. Available at: https://www.aaha.org/aaha-guidelines/life-stage-feline-2021/nutrition-and-weight-management/ (accessed 4 February 2022).

AAHA (American Animal Hospital Association) (2021b) Life stage checklists. Available at: https://www.aaha.org/aaha-guidelines/life-stage-canine-2019/life-stage-checklist/ (accessed 4 February 2022).

Alvarez, E.E., Schultz, K.K., Floerchinger, A.M. and Hull, J.L. (2022) Small animal general practitioners discuss nutrition infrequently despite assertion of indication, citing barriers. *Journal of the American Veterinary Medical Association,* 260(13), 1704–1710.

Baldwin, K., Bartges, J., Bufflington, T., Freeman, L.M., Grabow, M. *et al.* (2010) AAHA Nutritional Assessment Guidelines for Dogs and Cats. *Journal of the American Animal Hospital Association*, 46, 285–296.

Becvarova, I., Prochazka, D., Chandler, M.L. and Meyer, H. (2016) Nutrition education in European Veterinary Schools: Are European veterinary graduates competent in nutrition? *Journal of Veterinary Medical Education,* 43(4), 349–358.

Bergler, R., Wechsung, S., Kienzle, E., Hoff, T. and Dobenecker, B. (2016) Nutrition consultation in small animal practice – a field for specialized veterinarians. *Tierarztl Prax Ausg K Kleintiere Heimtiere,* 44, 5–14.

Blees, N.R., Vandendriessche, V.L., Corbee, R.J., Picavet, P. and Hesta, M. (2021) Nutritional consulting in regular veterinary practices in Belgium and the Netherlands. *Veterinary Medicine and Science*, 1–17.

Bruckner, I. and Handl, S. (2020) Survey on the role of nutrition in first-opinion practices in Austria and Germany: An evaluation of knowledge, preferences and need for further education. *Journal of Animal Physiology and Animal Nutrition,* 105 (Suppl. 2), 89–94.

Cardenas, D. (2013) Let not thy food be confused with thy medicine: The Hippocratic misquotation. *e-SPEN Journal,* 8(6), e260–e262.

Chandler, M. and Gunn-Moore, D. (2004) Nutritional status of canine and feline patients admitted to a referral veterinary internal medicine service. *Journal of Nutrition,* 134, 2050S–2052S.

Chandler, M. L. and Takashima, G. (2014) Veterinary concepts for the veterinary practitioner. *Veterinary Clinics of North America: Small Animal Practice,* 44, 645–666.

Churchill, J. and Ward, E. (2016) Communicating with pet owners about obesity: Roles of the veterinary health care team. *Veterinary Clinics of North America: Small Animal Practice,* 46, 899–911.

Cline, M.G., Burns, K.M., Coe, J.B., Downing, R., Durzi, T. *et al.* (2021) 2021 AAHA Nutrition and Weight Management Guidelines for Dogs and Cats. *Journal of the American Animal Hospital Association,* 57(4), 153–178.

Cornell, K.K. and Kopcha, M. (2007) Client-veterinarian communication: skills for client centered dialogue and shared decision making. *Veterinary Clinics of North America: Small Animal Practice,* 37(1), 37–47.

Creevy, K.E., Grady, J., Little, S.E., Moore, G.E., Groetzinger Strickler, B. *et al.* (2019) 2019 AAHA canine life stage guidelines. *Journal of the American Animal Hospital Association,* 55(6), 267–290.

Freeman, L., Becvarova, I., Cave, N., MacKay, C., Nguyen, P. *et al.* (2011) WSAVA Nutritional Assessment Guidelines. *Journal of Small Animal Practice,* 52(7), 385–396.

German, A. and Morgan, L. (2008) How often do veterinarians assess the bodyweight and body condition of dogs? *Veterinary Record,* 163, 503–505.

Johnson, L.N. and Linder, D. (2013) Making client communication appetising: talking with clients about nutrition. *The Veterinary Nurse,* 4(9), 542–548.

Kamleh, M., Khosa, D.K., Verbrugghe, A., Dewey, C.E. and Stone, E. (2020) A cross-sectional study of pet owners' attitudes and intentions towards nutritional guidance received from veterinarians. *Veterinary Record,* 187(12), e123.

Kealy, R.D., Lawler, D.F., Ballam, J.M., Mantz, S.L., Biery, D.N. *et al.* (2002) Effects of diet restriction on life span and age-related changes in dogs. *Journal of the American Veterinary Medical Association,* 220(9), 1315–1320.

Liu, D.T., Brown, D.C. and Silverstein, D.C. (2012) Early nutritional support is associated with decreased length of hospitalization in dogs with septic peritonitis: A retrospective study of 45 cases (2000–2009). *Journal of Veterinary Emergency and Critical Care,* 22(4), 453– 459.

Lumbis, R. and de Scally, M. (2020) Knowledge, attitudes and application of nutrition assessments by the veterinary health care team in small animal practice. *Journal of Small Animal Practice,* 61, 494–503.

MacMartin, C., Wheat, H.C., Coe, J.B. and Adams, C.L. (2015) Effect of question design on dietary information solicited during veterinarian-client interaction in companion animal practice in Ontario, Canada. *Journal of the American Veterinary Medical Association,* 246, 1203–1214.

Michel, K.E. (2009) Using a diet history to improve adherence to dietary recommendations. *Compendium on Continuing Education for the Practising Veterinarian,* 31(1), 22–24.

Michel, K.E., Willoughby, K.N., Abood, S.K., Fascetti, A.J., Fleeman, L.M. *et al.* (2008) Attitudes of pet owners toward pet foods and feeding management of cats and dogs. *Journal of the American Veterinary Medical Association,* 233(11), 1699–1703.

Mohr, A.J., Leisewitz, A.L., Jacobson, L.S., Steiner, J.M., Ruaux, C.G. *et al.* (2003) Effect of early enteral nutrition on intestinal permeability, intestinal protein loss, and outcome in dogs with severe parvoviral enteritis. *Journal of Veterinary Internal Medicine,* 17, 791–798.

Molina, J., Hervera, M., Manzanilla, E.G., Torrente, C. and Villaverde, C. (2018) Evaluation of the prevalence and risk factors for undernutrition in hospitalized dogs. *Frontiers in Veterinary Science,* 5, 205.

Quimby, J., Gowland, S., Carney, H.C., DePorter, T., Plummer, P. *et al.* (2021) 2021 AAHA/AAFP feline life stage guidelines. *Journal of the American Animal Hospital Association,* 57(2), 51–72.

Remillard, R.L., Darden, D.E., Michel, K.E., Marks, S.L., Buffington, C.A. *et al.* (2001) An investigation of the relationship between caloric intake and outcome in hospitalised dogs. *Veterinary Therapeutics,* 2, 301–310.

Rolph, N., Noble, P. and German, A. (2014) How often do primary care veterinarians record the overweight status of dogs? *Journal of Nutritional Science,* 3, E58.

Sallander, M. and Jaktlund, A. (2012/2013) Use of veterinary diets for dogs and cats hospitalized at a veterinary university clinic in Sweden. *The Veterinary Nurse,* 3, 638–644.

Santarossa, H.A., Parr, J.M. and Verbrugghe, A. (2018) Assessment of canine and feline body composition by veterinary healthcare teams in Ontario, Canada. *Canadian Veterinary Journal,* 59, 1280–1286.

Siebert, D., Schmidt, S., Hänse, M. and Coenen, M. (2016) The importance of nutrition counselling in veterinary practice. *Tierarztl Prax Ausg K Kleintiere Heimtiere,* 44, 158–162.

Vandendriessche, V.L., Hesta, M. and Picavet, P. (2017) First detailed nutritional survey in a referral companion animal population. *Journal of Animal Physiology and Animal Nutrition,* 101(S1), 4–14.

Villaverde, C. and Larsen, J. A. (2015) Nutritional Assessment. In: Silverstein, D. and Hopper, K. (eds) *Small Animal Critical Care Medicine,* 2nd edn. Saunders, St Louis, Missouri, pp. 673–676.

Wareham, K.J., Brennan, M.L. and Dean, R.S. (2019) Systematic review of the factors affecting cat and dog owner compliance with pharmaceutical treatment recommendations. *Veterinary Record,* 184(5), 154.

WSAVA (World Small Animal Veterinary Association) (2021) Global Nutrition Toolkit. Available at: https://wsava.org/wp-content/uploads/2021/04/WSAVA-Global-Nutrition-Toolkit-English.pdf (accessed 6 February 2022).

Yura, H. and Walsh, M. (1967) *The Nursing Process: Assessing, Planning, Implementing, and Evaluating.* Catholic University of America Press, Washington, USA.

Developing an interprofessional nutrition programme: It takes a team!

5

Tierney Kinnison

Abstract

Many facets of teamworking either contribute to a successful team and/or present challenges to collaboration. Hierarchy within a veterinary healthcare team (VHCT) is a natural occurrence due to the historic and legal differences between professions. Hierarchy can be used proactively to distribute advice in a practice regarding nutritional plans. Conversely, hierarchies may require flattening to allow individuals to seek information and advice from the most appropriate person, rather than an individual at the top of a profession-based hierarchy. Aspects of VHCTs' working lives can be used to enhance teamwork, for example consideration of ways to overcome temporal and spatial separation of groups, and the inclusion of carefully planned formal interprofessional infrastructure for communication. The benefits of a team arise due to the team members' differences (e.g. skills), and these differences should be valued. However, different perspectives and motivations for work, when misunderstood, can lead to challenges in interprofessional working.

The previous chapters have introduced the concept of the veterinary healthcare team (VHCT), with its interprofessional nature and state of dynamic evolution, alongside developments in understanding the importance of nutrition and the VHCT's role regarding what we have already seen described as the fifth vital sign. In this chapter, Chapter 5, through to Chapter 8, advice to enable a practice to develop and deliver an interprofessional nutrition programme tailored to that practice's context will be explored. Naturally the programmes developed by each reader of this chapter and their team are likely to vary depending on context and team/client requirements. However, some aspects of the programme may span different contexts – for example, previous chapters have recommended the creation of documentation outlining specific dietary recommendations and nutritional plans, developed in consultation with the caretaker, and provided at each consultation or on a pet's discharge from the hospital. These documents, therefore, can be tailored to the reader's context and the caregiver's situation.

© Rachel Lumbis and Tierney Kinnison 2023. *An Interprofessional Approach to Veterinary Nutrition* (R. Lumbis and T. Kinnison)
DOI: 10.1079/9781800621107.0005

This chapter focuses on attributes of a good, successful team, as well as challenges to interprofessional working, and how this understanding can be used to ensure the VHCT can provide the optimum nutritional care to its patients and advice to their caregivers. It is split into four sections: hierarchy, temporal and spatial nature of work, formal interprofessional infrastructure for communication, and perspectives and motivation.

Hierarchy

When considered as a way to describe the relationship between practice owners and managers, senior members of staff and junior members of staff, a hierarchy can be a useful and productive construct. A formalised structure taking into account seniority of positions and 'who has the information', for example, can allow people to know who to go to for help, as well as providing a map for information flow from senior staff to those for whom they are responsible (Kinnison *et al.*, 2016). Hierarchies may therefore provide natural and useful ways to organise a veterinary practice and a nutrition programme. Veterinarians are the only persons qualified to prescribe veterinary medicines, and they alongside suitably qualified persons (SQPs) hold the legal right to dispense prescriptions for animals. So, veterinarians initiate the process of prescribing. However, veterinary nurses (VNs), regardless of the SQP status, are typically in more frequent direct contact with an inpatient, and provide care in terms of feeding. In addition, they may have additional or alternative opportunities to speak to the patient's caretaker. Therefore, while maintaining the hierarchical structure of veterinarians and SQPs as the prescribers/dispensers, ensuring their veterinary nursing colleagues are kept abreast of their prescribing behaviours is important.

A veterinary practice hierarchy can also be conceptualised as one with influential individuals at the top, and those with less influence further down. In a study utilising social network analysis (SNA), it was shown that key influential people could be identified within veterinary practices via their comparatively increased network of interactions with others (Kinnison *et al.*, 2015a). Key people were primarily appointed leaders, with a professional role high in a traditional profession-based hierarchy – for example, veterinary directors/partners, head nurses and administrative managers. Informal or emergent leaders were rarer, although they did exist. In order to disseminate new processes, such as a nutritional programme, it may be important to identify your key people, ensure they are on board with the plan and enable them to communicate its details to their colleagues. However, care must be taken that these key people are not overloaded, as they are information brokers and must be provided with the time and processes to pass on their information and resources (Kinnison *et al.*, 2015a).

A contrasting perspective frequently regards hierarchies as in need of flattening due to the potential for professions higher up the hierarchy to stifle those below. For example, Heinrichs *et al.* (2012) advocate the use of situation, background, assessment and recommendation – SBAR – for communication about a patient's condition to flatten the hierarchy and improve communication in the US Navy, as well as in the medical professions, including obstetricians and nurses. Etherington *et al.* (2019) also discuss flattening hierarchies (of professions and status) to remove communication barriers and enable speaking up in operating rooms. The concept of speaking up for patient safety is explored in more depth in Chapter 7 which focuses on communication.

Hierarchies are linked to notions of power and status, and it is therefore quite usual for them to be built around the profession to which one belongs, rather than another aspect of oneself. In the veterinary field, the historic profession of the veterinarian heads the hierarchy, above their more recent professional colleagues, Registered Veterinary Nurses (RVNs), and other paraprofessionals and groups. This leads to the likely occurrence of individuals seeking help, advice and support from those higher up in the traditional hierarchy, even if that person is not the ideal individual with regard to knowledge/skills. The SNA research highlighted above described the existence of this profession-based hierarchy in veterinary practices (Kinnison *et al.*, 2015a). Four interactions were reported from this study: gaining information, asking for advice, problem solving and being influenced by another. The density of each type of interaction for veterinarians was higher with other veterinarians than with VNs, meaning that veterinarians interacted with each other more than any other group. In contrast, the density of each type of interaction for VNs was similar with both veterinarians and other VNs. In addition, reciprocity scores showed that VNs who communicated with a veterinarian regarding one of the four types of interactions may not experience reciprocation of the behaviour. In simple terms, I ask you for help and advice, but you don't ask me. Together, the one-way lack of reciprocation and the density scores indicate the existence of the traditional hierarchical structure between veterinarians and VNs (Kinnison *et al.*, 2015a). This reflects homophily, the desire to interact with those like ourselves, and may be at odds with seeking out the right individual with the required experience and knowledge. However, examples of information- and advice-seeking based on knowledge, rather than simply the profession to which an individual belongs, were also frequently seen in the wider parts of this veterinary interprofessional study, and suggest a complex and fluid hierarchy of interactions (Kinnison *et al.*, 2016). This can be termed an 'experience-based hierarchy', and such experienced-based hierarchies have also been explored in interactions between doctors and nurses on surgical wards, whereby it was seen as natural and healthy for doctors to rely on experienced nurses; however, it was also noted that those lacking experience from any profession may struggle to express views and have an influence (Vatn and Dahl, 2022).

A further finding from the SNA study mentioned above was that there is an association between being social with a colleague outside of work and all four interactions studied (receiving information, asking for advice, problem solving and being influenced by another) (Kinnison, *et al.*, 2015a). This suggests that to reduce a potentially negative, stifling hierarchy, and to promote interprofessional collaboration, endeavours to facilitate the social nature of a practice team may be valuable.

Temporal and spatial nature of work

It may seem like common sense, but empirical research has identified that interactions are easier when individuals share a space at the same time. In veterinary practices, pictorial representation of interactions between individuals identified a lack of resource-sharing (information, advice etc.) between branches, thus limiting the ability to be a cohesive team (Kinnison *et al.*, 2015b). The 'sociogram' shown in Fig. 5.1 is an example of this pictorial representation of interactions. In this case, the interaction was problem-solving with another person. All members of a practice team were asked to identify with whom they problem solve, and via computer software, a sociogram was automatically created to demonstrate the best fit to the data. This sociogram

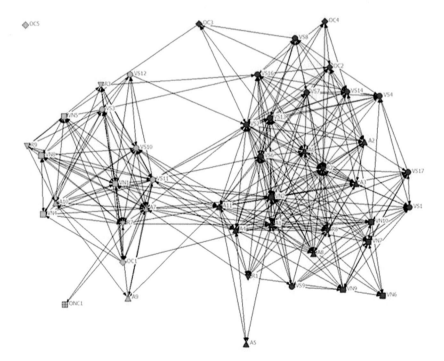

Fig. 5.1. Sociogram of 'Practice code 9', displaying the interaction of problem-solving. Colours indicate the two branches of the practice. Shapes indicate professions (square = RVN, circle = veterinarian, down triangle = receptionist, up triangle = administrator, diamond = other). Author's own figure.

shows people as 'nodes' (dots), with the shape of the node determined by their profession (e.g. square = RVN) and their colour determined by the branch to which they belong. In this instance, the sociogram clearly shows the divide between the two branches for the interaction 'problem-solving', and this divide in interactions was mirrored for receiving information, receiving advice and being influenced by another.

For a new nutritional programme to be successfully implemented into a practice with multiple branches, therefore, extra effort will be required to ensure the programme is communicated and supported sufficiently. This is proposed as an ideal opportunity to use the key, influential people, as discussed earlier, as they are frequently individuals who can span boundaries such as branch locations as well as professions. Individuals who work across branches would also be valuable in ensuring all branches are following the agreed protocols. The idea of a 'nutrition champion' who will develop as an emergent key person (leader) in nutrition in the practice is further explored in Chapter 8.

In addition, observational research as part of this wider veterinary research project identified challenges from the temporal organisation of work. There was a limited time within each day whereby veterinarians and VNs were actually together and had the opportunity to speak at any length. Time together primarily occurred during surgery, which becomes a focal point for conversations about more than just the patient at hand. In some practices, the existence of branch practices which did not have a veterinarian on site for several hours throughout the day were noted (Kinnison *et al.*, 2016). To address temporal and spatial issues, research in human healthcare has investigated the use of smartphones, and while access to emails for non-urgent information and calls for urgent access to clinicians was generally favoured, there was some dissatisfaction, including with appropriate use of the tools (Lo *et al.*, 2012).

In primary healthcare settings in Canada, interprofessional communication was also seen to be impacted by time and space; however, there were differing experiences depending on the context, such as physical layouts of clinical space (Oandasan *et al.*, 2009). This suggests there is unlikely to be a one size fits all approach to interprofessional collaboration in a nutritional programme, and that individual practices will need to work together to develop the optimum approach for their setting. Further research has suggested that it is not only the issues of literal time and space, but also cultural aspects of these factors, including feelings of territoriality by one profession over a certain area, creating perceived spatial boundaries, and resulting in recommendations to also explore team and professional cultures in addition to physical locations (Fernando *et al.*, 2016).

Formal interprofessional infrastructure for communication

Seemingly another factor supported by common sense, having formal, scheduled interprofessional meetings, enables all members of staff to feel that their group is represented, valued and has a voice in decision-making. Examples include management meetings which include appropriately selected nominees from different categories of practice staff, so all professions and groups are indeed represented (Kinnison *et al.*, 2016), and nutritional standards consensus meetings including all professions, as explored in Chapter 8. As such, any meeting whereby a new nutritional programme is introduced should aim to include representation from all professions and occupations who will be involved in its delivery, or are required to be aware of its existence, so that there can be shared understanding and true team ownership of new programmes. This is likely to include all groups: veterinarians, VNs, receptionists and administrators such as practice managers.

Frequent interprofessional meetings, as well as daily rounds, are not only useful for disseminating information effectively, but can also be used to enable the team to identify when a collaborative approach to a case is necessary, and how this could be developed, as reported in the hospitalised care of older adults (Dahlke *et al.*, 2020). In a systematic review of interprofessional collaboration in healthcare, it was concluded that interprofessional meetings may slightly improve the team's adherence to recommended practices and that interprofessional rounds may slightly improve the use of healthcare resources, such as length of stay and cost to patients. However, the evidence had low certainty and was contradictory between included studies (Reeves *et al.*, 2017). This suggests further research is required to evaluate the best way to use interprofessional meetings.

It is acknowledged that almost any professional in any profession will not be keen on more meetings. In addition, scheduling meetings which are inclusive of individuals from all professions has logistical challenges. Therefore, while the empirical advice is in favour of the benefits of structured interprofessional meetings, how this will actually be implemented into a veterinary practice will depend on the context.

Perspectives and motivation

Different professions, and of course even different individuals within a profession, will have different perspectives on a nutritional case. It is these differences that are actually the reason why a team is often better than an individual at approaching a complex problem. As explored in Chapter 2, distributed cognition (Hutchins, 1995) allows a team to have a wide range of knowledge and understanding, without any one individual needing to know everything. This knowledge can then provide different perspectives, which can help a team come to the best decision for the patient and its caretaker.

In the veterinary interprofessional research cited throughout this chapter, different perspectives between veterinarian partners and administrators were often highlighted regarding the business aspects of the practice (Kinnison *et al.*, 2016). However, the value of different perspectives equally applies to the clinical professions, with veterinarians and VNs able to benefit from each other's differing undergraduate education, continuing professional development, past working experiences, and current knowledge and awareness. Nutrition of patients is relevant to the healthcare provided by both clinical professions, and VNs are in a prime position to offer individual insights into inpatients in their care with regard to nutritional plans, and these perspectives should be sought and listened to. In order for this to occur, a solid foundation of trust is required between the professions, and this is explored further in Chapter 6.

While it is the differences between groups which makes interprofessional working so successful, it is also a source of challenges when working together. One aspect of this is the underlying motivation for an individual's actions. Where the motivation is different, and especially where it is not understood between individuals, tensions in work may emerge. For example, interview research has suggested that VNs' primary motivation for their actions at work is linked to the animal, in terms of overall healthcare, animal welfare and being an advocate for the animal, followed by consideration for the client (Kinnison *et al.*, 2016). This was proposed as being in contrast to a veterinarian's primary motivation for their actions at work, which related more closely to clinical treatment of conditions affecting the patient and practice management, and to receptionists' motivation whose focus was primarily on the client (Kinnison *et al.*, 2016). These competing stakeholders, and the differing directions in which the professions find themselves pulled, may result in competing actions of the individuals within the team and tensions if an individual's desired action is not followed. To address these potential challenges, open communication regarding the reasons for underlying actions would be beneficial, although it is acknowledged that, at least at first, this will take additional time.

While it is important to raise these differing primary motivations, the potential issues they may cause, and an idea for ways to address them, there is a concern that when phrased as simply as this, some professions may take offence, and this may worsen interprofessional relations. It is paramount to explain that the motivations outlined here were identified as the *primary* orientations, and not the *only* motivations. It does not suggest that veterinarians do not care for the overall health of their patients. Nor does it suggest that VNs have no interest in the business side of practice, or that receptionists are not concerned with the patients that walk through the front door. At any one time, any individual within a veterinary practice is working for multiple stakeholders, and while naturally working for the benefit of all, they may on occasion have to focus their attention on one. It is these times that warrant further thought and action plans to allow shared decision-making between the team and the caretaker for the ultimate benefit of the patient. This should involve open communication which allows each professional and the caretaker to explain and explore their expectations, desired pathways for progress and the reasoning behind these feelings.

In summary

A VHCT works through balancing the demands of several stakeholders, including the patient, caregiver, practice, and needs of the team and society. In order to work as a good interprofessional team, capable of delivering effective and patient-centred nutritional care, several aspects of practice should be considered. These include the following: hierarchy – utilising useful hierarchies and flattening others to enable individuals to seek advice from the best person possible; temporal and spatial nature of work – cultivating a culture and a physical location whereby the VHCT can be together to better enable communication and collaboration; formal interprofessional infrastructure – incorporation of inclusive meetings to aid communication and identification of cases for interprofessional working; perspectives and motivation – acknowledgement and celebration of our differences, through open communication, regarding motivation, in order to better understand each other's desired plans for patient care.

References

Dahlke, S., Hunter, K.F., Reshef Kalogirou, M., Negrin, K., Fox, M. *et al.* (2020) Perspectives about interprofessional collaboration and patient-centred care. *Canadian Journal on Aging*, 39(3), 443–455.

Etherington, N., Wu, M., Cheng-Boivin, O., Larrigan, S. and Boet, S. (2019) Interprofessional communication in the operating room: a narrative review to advance research and practice. *Canadian Journal of Anesthesia*, 66(10), 1251–1260.

Fernando, O., Coburn, N.G., Nathens, A.B. Hallet, J., Ahmed, N. *et al.* (2016) Interprofessional communication between surgery trainees and nurses in the inpatient wards: Why time and space matter. *Journal of Interprofessional Care*, 30(5), 567–573.

Heinrichs, W.L., Bauman, E. and Dev, P. (2012) SBAR 'flattens the hierarchy' among caregivers. *Studies in Health Technology and Informatics*, 173, 175–182.

Hutchins, E. (1995) *Cognition in the Wild*. Massachusetts Institute of Technology, Cambridge, MA.

Kinnison, T., Guile, D. and May, S.A. (2015a) Veterinary team interactions, part 2: The personal effect. *Veterinary Record*, 177(21), 541.

Kinnison, T., May, S.A., Guile, D. (2015b) Veterinary team interactions, part 1: The practice effect. *Veterinary Record*, 177(16), 419.

Kinnison, T., Guile, D. and May, S.A. (2016) The case of veterinary interprofessional practice: From one health to a world of its own. *Journal of Interprofessional Education and Practice*, 4, 51–57.

Lo, V., Wu, R.C., Morra, D., Lee, L. and Reeves, S. (2012) The use of smartphones in general and internal medicine units: A boon or a bane to the promotion of interprofessional collaboration?. *Journal of Interprofessional Care*, 26(4), 276–282.

Oandasan, I.F, Gotlib Conn, L., Lingard, L., Karim, A., Jakubovicz, D. *et al.* (2009) The impact of space and time on interprofessional teamwork in Canadian primary health care settings: Implications for health care reform. *Primary Health Care Research and Development*, 10(2), 151–162.

Reeves, S., Pelone, F., Harrison, R., Goldman, J. and Zwarenstein, M. (2017) Interprofessional collaboration to improve professional practice and healthcare outcomes. The Cochrane database of systematic reviews, 6(6), CD000072.

Vatn, L. and Dahl, B.M. (2022) Interprofessional collaboration between nurses and doctors for treating patients in surgical wards. *Journal of Interprofessional Care*, 36(2), 186–194.

Developing an interprofessional nutrition programme: Trust, values and ethics

Rachel Lumbis

6

Abstract

Public awareness of the importance of optimal nutrition to health and wellbeing is growing and caretakers are increasingly focusing on their pets' nutrition. However, there is common misinformation and misperceptions surrounding nutrition and a growing mistrust of commercially produced pet food, contributing to inappropriate or imbalanced nutrition and undue harm to pets. Interactions between veterinary practices and clients have also become increasingly transactional, particularly when discussing nutrition, resulting in a growing scepticism and cynicism of veterinarians' motivations. Pet caregiver decisions are often heavily informed by subconscious influences, including personal experience, opinions, values and beliefs, and are frequently made before considering alternative courses of action (Faulkner, 2013). Consequently, the relationship between veterinary professionals and pet caretakers needs to be stronger than ever, with establishment of trust and rapport proving crucial. This chapter will review the subconscious influences on dietary-related decision-making and purchasing choices, provide strategies to build client confidence and trust, and identify ways to help clients understand the value behind nutritional recommendations.

The importance of trust, values and ethics

According to the quote attributed to Hippocrates, 'Science is the father of knowledge, but opinion breeds ignorance'. As already highlighted in Chapter 3, sound scientific evidence is regarded as paramount, yet nutrition-related fads, myths and misconceptions are widespread. Popular sources of dietary-related advice such as the internet, social media, breeders, friends, family members and pet store workers can prove compelling to pet caretakers yet, while usually well-intentioned, the advice and information offered by these sources is often unfounded and subject to bias (Chandler, 2018). Personal experience, beliefs and opinion are highly subjective and

DOI: 10.1079/9781800621107.0006

affected by cognitive bias, particularly the Dunning-Kruger effect, determining trust and actions (Chandler, 2018).

Trust

With a growing mistrust of commercial pet foods, either because of their composition, processing or a perceived corrupt industry (Michel *et al.*, 2008), trust is one of the many determinants that influences caretakers' pet food purchase and feeding management. Trust is also one of the most fundamental qualities of human relationships and is integral to honing and maintaining effective relationships with clients and pet caretakers, as well as colleagues. Bonded clients have a higher level of trust for veterinary care and recommendations, resulting in the provision of better care and the chance of a longer and happier life for patients (Hauser, 2022).

Grand *et al.* (2013) identified professionalism and technical candour, in addition to perceived competence, as key indicators of veterinarian trustworthiness according to standardised clients. A small-scale simulation study by Tuisku *et al.* (2018) identified that emotional, rather than scarce or factual, provision of information, a direct gaze and body direction and an emotional, rather than routine, style of behaviour positively influenced clients' evaluation of the expertise and trustworthiness of the veterinarian. Further strategies to build the confidence and trust of clients include:

- Provide a warm, open and friendly welcome and show that you care about the pet and their caretaker.
- Make a connection, for example, by complimenting the caretaker on their pet.
- Ensure that you practise 'active listening' when communicating with clients and gain clarification when necessary. Ensure that you understand their objectives for their pet and any concerns they have. Concerns often relate to four Ps – pain, prognosis, price and practicalities – all of which must be addressed when making decisions (Faulkner, 2013).
- Involve caretakers in the care and treatment of their pet, including the setting of goals.
- Emphasise to caretakers that the nutritional recommendation is being made in the best interests of their pet.
- Be empathetic to the client's perspective – this doesn't mean you necessarily have to agree with, or support this, but empathy is critical to building trust in the veterinary healthcare team (VHCT)–client relationship.
- Maintain comprehensive medical records and ensure effective interprofessional communication and standardised practice protocols.
- Demonstrate sincerity, honesty and integrity – admit to any uncertainty or error.
- Keep to your word and follow through with assurances.

- Encourage younger or more reserved members of the team to build relationships with clients by telling the client everything they are doing to the pet (Felsted, 2012). For example, 'I am going to assess Nelson's body condition now by feeling his chest and ribs and by checking for a tummy tuck and waistline.'
- Be patient – building trust and rapport with clients can take time and continuity.

As outlined in Chapter 3, clients frequently prioritise and rely upon pet health information received from non-veterinary sources, especially those who have mistrust in commercially produced pet food, potentially resulting in reduced client–veterinarian engagement. This is a particular challenge in relation to clients seeking information about nutrition (Janke *et al.*, 2021). Yet the veterinarian is commonly reported as the primary source of nutrition information among pet caretakers (Michel *et al.*, 2008; Prata, 2022) who also have a high level of trust in veterinarians for nutrition advice (Kamleh *et al.*, 2020). Greater trust and intentions towards veterinary-sourced nutrition information and advice is also associated with higher perceived effectiveness of veterinary nutrition care (Kamleh *et al.*, 2020). Generating trust and rapport with clients is therefore crucial to establishing the VHCT as the primary source of nutritional advice. It can also influence clients' attitudes toward, and perceptions of, veterinarians and the veterinary profession, which can significantly influence the likelihood of future visits (Grand *et al.*, 2013).

Over recent years, the interactions between veterinary practices and clients have become increasingly transactional. Subsequently, pet caretakers have grown increasingly sceptical and cynical of the motives of the VHCT, resulting in reduced collaboration and compliance. Janke *et al.* (2021) revealed that pet caretakers feel pressured and/or have a lack of involvement in the decision-making process and believe that veterinarians' intentions and a lack of options are commonly associated with veterinarians' financial motivations. This was found to be particularly relevant when discussing nutrition. Participants questioned the veterinarian's motivations around the recommendation for, and sale of, pet food and were convinced that the veterinarian promoted a particular brand of food because it resulted in personal gain, rather than letting the client make the 'most informed decision' (Janke *et al.*, 2021, p. 11). Likewise, Kamleh *et al.* (2020) found that first-year veterinary students and pre-veterinary students felt similar conflict about the motives behind veterinarians' dietary recommendations, with some perceiving this to be biased and/or influenced by financial incentives. Describing dietary options on a higher order level that involves more than just the simple recommendation of brand or product names can help to reduce such suspicion, as can educating caretakers about their options so an informed decision can be made (MacMartin *et al.*, 2018). A shared decision-making approach when making dietary changes is further predicted to help reduce clients' mistrust of veterinarians (Janke *et al.*, 2021) and potentially also commercially produced pet food.

A relationship exists between satisfaction and loyalty and, while one does not always have a direct effect on the other, both are influenced by several factors including trust, value, commitment and communication (Brown, 2018). In many veterinary practices, clients are no longer loyal to one veterinarian, but rather to the entire VHCT (Prendergast, 2016). This is particularly pertinent in relation to the provision of nutritional recommendations and care, in which the entire team plays a key role. Predictors of pet–caretaker trust in the veterinarian were examined by Brown (2018). Customer service and communication skills of veterinary technicians significantly predicted trust in the veterinarian, as did satisfaction with communication from the veterinarian, and customer service and communication skills from reception staff. Effective communication skills and the VHCT's ability to clearly explain the reasons for their recommendations drives clients' perceptions of the value and quality of care (Lue *et al.*, 2008). Such findings emphasise the importance of ensuring that each team member provides a positive communication experience with clients and a seamless service. Pet caretakers who are satisfied with communication from staff members are nearly twice as likely to be behaviourally loyal, and the likelihood of such loyalty improves when the same veterinarian is seen and when a veterinary consultation is the primary source for healthcare questions (Brown, 2018). Pairing up a client with specific members of the VHCT can help to ensure continuity and consistency and build a relationship that feels personal rather than transactional. Benefits of pet caretakers seeing and speaking to the same veterinary professionals and client support staff are acknowledged by Felsted (2012) and include:

1. Knowledge. The creation of a knowledge relationship, whereby the veterinary professional builds a comprehensive understanding of the pet's medical history and behaviour, as well as an appreciation of the caretaker's circumstances, lifestyle, preferences and concerns. This helps provide personalised and consistent recommendations and, thus, increases the likelihood of compliance (Hansen, 2021).
2. Trust. Continuity helps to build a bond between veterinary professional, caretaker and pet, resulting in a higher likelihood of a trusting relationship. Subsequently, caretakers' acceptance of recommendations and compliance is more likely, as is their promotion of the veterinary practice to friends, family members and colleagues.
3. Value. Treating veterinarians and veterinary nurses as interchangeable cogs in the relationship between the practice, pet and caretaker could devalue their importance to the caretaker.

Values

Values are subjectively held beliefs and deep-rooted abstract motivations that are shaped from an early age and become increasingly permanent, giving significance to a person's life (Rokeach, 1973). Values reflect what is most important to an individual and, together with thoughts and feelings, influence mind-set. They also define non-negotiable behaviours and are guiding forces behind personal priorities, decision-making, perceptions and attitudes. Examples of value types include ethical/moral, doctrinal/ideological (such as religious/political), social and aesthetic.

A value system, or set, functions at individual and organisational levels (Feather, 1995), with values expressed in a hierarchical order, determining the priority, or perceived importance, of each value (Tuulik *et al.*, 2016) and thus its influence on behaviour. A value is distinguished by the underlying goal or motivation that it expresses and what is important to one individual may not be to another.

There are many typologies of values, the aim of which is to categorise types of values and to limit the number of words used to express values (Tuulik *et al.*, 2016). One of the most established typologies of individual values is the Rokeach Value Survey (Rokeach, 1973) which lists terminal or intrinsic values (desirable end-states of existence), such as equality and happiness, and instrumental values (preferable modes of conduct), such as honesty and capability. Values may also be expressed according to different levels, demonstrating which individual values coincide with those held by others (Tuulik *et al.*, 2016).

Explaining the value of proactive care

The bond between veterinary practice (and VHCT), client and pet is heavily influenced by communication, pet interaction, ability to educate and providing only products and services the pet needs (Gerrard, 2015; Lue *et al.*, 2008). The stronger the caretaker–pet bond, the greater the likelihood that clients will have a higher perception of value, seek high quality care, be more willing to follow veterinary recommendations and be less sensitive to the price of care (Lue *et al.*, 2008). Clients need to believe that the aim of the VHCT is to get their pet as well as possible, as quickly as possible, as easily as possible and as cheaply as possible. Yet, while financial constraints are not the principal reason for poor uptake of veterinary services and products (Little, 2013), the cost of veterinary services is a leading reason for a client to leave a veterinary practice (Brown, 2018) and is uncommonly discussed in companion animal practice (Groves *et al.*, 2022).

In a survey by Volk *et al.* (2011), a reported 36% of caretakers only take a pet to the veterinarian to have vaccinations, 32% stated they only take their pet if it becomes sick, and 24% believed that routine examinations are unnecessary. According to a current US-based study, nearly half of dog (49%) and cat (44%) caretakers attend an annual veterinary visit for preventative pet healthcare, but a respective 16% and 36% fail to participate in any of the actions presented (Bir *et al.*, 2020). The more recent American Veterinary Medical

Association (AVMA) survey of pet and caretaker demographics indicated that a respective 24% and 35% of dog and cat caretakers don't seek annual health-care for their pets, primarily due to a lack of perceived value of this care and affordability (Hauser, 2022). One reason attributed to this disconnect is mis-alignment between the VHCT and client's understanding of what constitutes preventative care. Caretakers perceive this care to be, largely, self-driven, for example, through the provision of diet, exercise and socialisation, with some involvement from trusted sources including groomers, breeders, trainers and day-care providers, but little contribution made by the VHCT. As a result, veterinary preventative healthcare is viewed as a service – for example, the administration of vaccinations and parasite prevention treatment, and inter-actions with veterinarians are increasingly seen as transactional (Banfield Pet Hospital, 2015). Encouraging routine and regular pet visits to the veterinary practice facilitates the development of a deeper relationship between caretaker, pet and VHCT. It can also help to expand the role of the VHCT beyond the scope of medical provider, enabling the provision of guidance in other important areas of proactive care, such as diet, exercise, behaviour and the selection of pet products (Hansen, 2021).

Suggestions of how the VHCT can help clients to understand the value behind clinical recommendations are offered by Hauser (2022) and include:

- Take time to explore a caretaker's expectations, alongside a discussion regarding their pet's health, diet, behaviour, breed-specific and life-stage needs. This can build a stronger relationship and promote the need for pre-ventative care and appropriate diet choices throughout every stage of the pet's life (Banfield Pet Hospital, 2015).
- Enquire about caretakers' short and long-term goals for their pet's health (including diet) and perceived barriers to optimal pet health and nutrition to help tailor the appointment to meet clients' needs. This is critical to rela-tionship-building and client buy-in.
- Have candid conversations with clients about their fears regarding (nutritional) recommendations and use empathetic questioning. For example:
  - What concerns you about the nutritional recommendations being presented?
  - What would help you to be more comfortable with the nutritional recommendation?
  - What can we do to support you in making the recommended change to Buster's diet?
- Prevent disconnects when explaining the value and benefits of a (nutri-tional) recommendation. Clients expect options and will choose the one that most closely aligns to their own beliefs and values. If the views of the VHCT and client are misaligned, this could result in a negative emotional outcome (Faulkner, 2013). Ultimately, clients want their decisions to be respected and don't want to be judged or made to feel guilty.

Clients' general lack of understanding of the value of routine and preventative care and affordability, together with confusion around veterinary recommendations and fear of the unknown can break the bond with a veterinary practice and result in clients declining care and treatment of their pets (Nolen, 2021; Hauser, 2022). The totality of care that a pet requires must be fully explained in a way in which the pet caretaker understands and values (Brown, 2018) with communication of the cost framed in relation to the benefits offered to the pet's future health and wellbeing (Groves *et al.*, 2022).

The influence of value proposition in making dietary decisions

Values are a framework for vision and what we do. They are a central component of each individual and their personality and are critical motivators of personal behaviours and attitudes. How can the VHCT instil that a pet's healthcare, including diet, is as important to its caretaker as, for example, buying a luxury coffee every day or going to a pub, bar or restaurant every weekend? This is a value proposition.

A value proposition is a widely used concept, particularly in business and marketing, and consists of a statement, typically developed as part of a broader marketing strategy, communicating how a company aims to provide value and benefits to its customers through its services or products (Payne *et al.*, 2017). In the veterinary industry, it can help to identify how one practice differs from other local competitors and why it should be the practice of choice for pet caretakers (Felsted, 2012), ultimately determining how clients view a practice (Lewis, 2017). Clients' assessment of value is based on personal perception of what is given and received. Given that value can be created and perceived through multiple elements, including price, quality, location and convenience (Hassan, 2012), clients' perceptions and expectations will differ, making value proposition highly individual and situational (Cooper *et al.*, 2022). It is therefore essential to consider the perspectives of clients. Involving employees in the development of value propositions is also crucial to help them understand what you want the practice to represent, identify what role they play in doing that and provide a sense of ownership in the delivery (Lewis, 2017, p. 159). A well designed marketing strategy can help to ensure clear communication of the value proposition, thus enhancing the client-perceived value and increasing the likelihood of positive attitudinal and behavioural outcomes as well as financial success of the business (Arslanagic-Kalajdzic and Zabkar, 2015). Guidance on how to construct value propositions is offered by Lewis (2017).

Discussing diet and nutrition at every veterinary visit can enhance clients' understanding and attitudes toward veterinary care and highlight the support available from the VHCT in decision-making (Hansen, 2021). However, people hold their own values and beliefs with a high degree of conviction that they are 'right', and pet caretakers will therefore gravitate towards sources of information most closely aligned to these, even if they are inaccurate and misinformed. What starts as one person's opinion can easily become widely accepted and reversing a fashionable theory can then prove to be both difficult and unpopular

(McNeill, 2018). Not all clients rate highly the importance of optimal diet and nutrition for their pet or the knowledge and expertise of the VHCT. It is therefore important to understand the values, beliefs and value proposition of nutrition as perceived by pet caretakers so that veterinary services and products can be designed and delivered in alignment. It is also important to consider those of the company and its employees. Organisational values are key to developing and driving the culture of the workplace and are closely linked to leadership and motivation of the employees (Tuulik *et al.*, 2016). Every employee brings personal values to an organisation and veterinary practices can devise their own value set, or system, by ordering and prioritising their own set of principles, standards or desirable qualities that are congruent with their value propositions and client service and experience. Staff members' customer service skills is a commonly cited reason for pet caregivers leaving a veterinary practice, therefore understanding what clients want and expect should be a priority for every veterinary practice (Brown, 2018).

As discussed in Chapter 3, food provision is considered a primary means of expressing care and so the VHCT should focus diet-related marketing and nutrition conversations on the bond between caretaker, pet and VHCT. In a study by Lue *et al.*, (2008), a correlation was found between caretakers who were strongly bonded to their pet and those that fed specialty foods, including prescription, life stage and premium diets. Yet pet food, including prescription diets, doesn't have to be procured from the veterinary practice. Lower prices and convenience drive the value proposition in e-commerce channels (Hansen, 2021), contributing to a lack of caretaker reliance on the veterinary practice and decreases in revenue (Bir *et al.*, 2020). The way caretakers perceive the effectiveness of veterinary nutrition care is also influenced by their chosen supplier of pet food, potentially due to the likelihood of receiving a conflicting nutrition recommendation from a non-veterinary source, such as a pet shop (Kamleh *et al.*, 2020). This needs to be considered when conducting nutrition conversations in a clinical setting.

Educating clients about the rationale behind the recommendation(s) being made and ensuring their understanding of, and concordance with, this will build trust, acceptance, perception of the value of the nutrition services being offered, and a willingness to pay (Prendergast, 2016). As outlined by Volk *et al.* (2011), regular visits to the veterinary practice are also more likely if caretakers understand the:

- value of the recommendation in terms of how it will benefit their pet's health and wellbeing
- economic benefits to themselves (e.g. the avoidance of expensive future treatment).
- need for, and value of, routine preventative health, or wellness, examinations (including frequent nutritional assessments) at every stage of their pet's life.

Ultimately, it is important to understand how the various (diet-related) products and (nutrition) services that can or could be offered, and your perceived needs of clients, connect with what clients want (Lewis, 2017).

Ethics

Ethics are considered beliefs or principles that govern right from wrong and are often emotive, making conversations challenging (Morgan and McDonald, 2007). Ethics-based food choices and dietary-related decisions are often defined by personal values (intrinsic motivators), morals (personal belief of what is good) and principles (personal belief of what is right) (Food Ethics Council, 2022). Ethical concerns that often influence purchasing decisions include:

- environmental impact
- animal welfare
- human rights and welfare
- food safety
- food production process – for example, genetic modification.

A moral dilemma is defined by Morgan and McDonald (2007) as a conflict between responsibilities or obligations of exactly equal moral weight and can occur when there are competing responsibilities with no obvious prioritisation. The feeding of companion animals is associated with two key obligations – the responsibility of caretakers to feed pets an appropriate diet and a simultaneous compulsion to avoid feeding a diet which conflicts with their duties to others (Milburn, 2016). People who avoid eating animals are more likely to be pet caretakers, with ethically motivated meat abstainers likely to have a greater number of companion animals than those motivated by health concerns or a combination of ethical and health concerns (Rothgerber, 2013). A moral dilemma may arise when they are faced with feeding animal products to their omnivorous dogs and carnivorous cats (Dodd *et al.*, 2019). As obligate carnivores, the provision of a vegan diet for cats has been considered particularly problematic and potentially questionable in terms of nutritional adequacy (Michel, 2006; Zafalon *et al.*, 2020). For vegan and ethical meat abstaining caretakers, this presents a conflict of two sacred values: protecting the wellbeing of their pet and protecting the wellbeing of other animals and the environment. While for health-motivated, meat abstaining caretakers, the moral problem is more likely to be simplified as their primary concern is the health of their pet with less or no regard for the impact on other animals or the environment (Rothgerber, 2013).

Although vegetarianism and veganism are often grouped together in nutritional and psychological investigations, Rosenfield (2019) identified a difference in identity profiles which should be considered when communicating with clients from each dietarian group. Key findings in vegans compared to vegetarians include:

- viewing diet as being more connected and central to identity
- having higher private regard and greater pride taken in their diet
- perceived lower public regard and a greater feeling of stigmatism for following a vegan diet
- possessing stronger dietary motivations
- judging omnivorous dieters more harshly.

Ethical dilemmas can also arise in nutrition support situations (Ferrie, 2006) and, due to their highly emotive nature, can prove challenging, particularly for a VHCT that practises evidence-based veterinary medicine. As identified by Ferrie (2006, p. 113), 'the emotional and personal nature of ethical decision making can present difficulties, and conflict can arise when people have different ethical perspectives'. When communicating about pet food decisions and nutritional support, it is essential for the VHCT to understand caretakers' values and ethical principles to ensure alignment of nutritional and other veterinary recommendations. Factors such as culture can have a key influence on the foods that individuals include in and exclude from their diet, and potentially that of their pets, as well as the way it is prepared. It is also important to distinguish between dietarian groups to better appreciate differences in how people think, feel, and behave regarding animal products (Rosenfield, 2019). For clients seeking further information about ethical consumerism in relation to pet food production and diet choices, appropriate signposting should be provided to trusted resources such as https://www.ethicalconsumer.org, as well as to veterinary-recommended nutrition-related resources, examples of which are outlined in Chapter 3. Tips for managing potentially controversial and contentious conversations can be found in Chapter 7. The application of an ethical theory can help guide ethical decision-making and determine the interrelationships and consequences of all factors and decisions (Fornari, 2015). These include:

- **consequentialism theories**, for example utilitarianism, which determine whether an action is good or bad according to its outcome, or consequences
- **non-consequentialism theories**, for example deontology, that consider actions to be determined by rules and therefore right or wrong, irrespective of the outcome, or consequences
- **animal rights philosophy**, whereby animals are considered equal to humans, are recognised to have an inherent worth and should never be used as a means to an end
- **virtue ethics and ethics of care**, involving an individualised approach to care, using individual, subjective, and emotional response as a guide to action
- **the biomedical ethical theory of Beauchamp and Childress**, which is grounded in four key healthcare principles; autonomy (being able to act autonomously), non-maleficence (do no harm), beneficence (promotion of good) and justice (fair, equitable, and appropriate treatment).

In addition, Ferrie (2006) recommends the adoption of a step-by-step approach to resolving ethical issues:

1. Distinctly clarify the relevant question, or questions.
2. Establish any relevant guidelines, for example, a defined ethical stance or existing guidelines or codes of conduct.
3. Gather objective information, for example, the caretaker's feelings about food and nutritional support and the results of their pet's nutritional assessment.

4. Define key terms, for example, quality of life.

5. Consider all information and discuss with all stakeholders. This should include the use of analogies and consideration of the outcome of past, similar patient scenarios; listing all options and potential outcomes; and exploring the beliefs and feelings of each stakeholder.

Beliefs can be unacknowledged influences on pet caretakers' decision-making, causing conflict between different ethical perspectives. Ensuring that all members of the VHCT have an awareness of ethical issues can help in defining the source of the conflict and finding a resolution.

In summary

A wide range of intrinsic and extrinsic factors influence pet caregivers' decision-making and dietary choices. Despite being a commonly cited source of information about pet care and nutrition, not all clients trust the VHCT and instead prioritise the use of the alternative sources of information. This, together with the increasing popularity of unconventional diets and a distrust of commercially produced pet food, increases the risk of feeding a nutritionally inadequate and imbalanced diet, with severe and detrimental consequences to pet health and wellbeing. Understanding the context for clients' pet feeding behaviour, alongside considering and respecting personal values, beliefs, concerns and goals, is essential for achieving consensus and concordance in relation to nutritional, and other veterinary, recommendations.

References

Arslanagic-Kalajdzic, M. and Zabkar, V. (2015) The external effect of marketing accountability in business relationships: Exploring the role of customer perceived value. *Industrial Marketing Management*, 46, 83–97.

Banfield Pet Hospital (2015) A guide to improving preventative care for pets. Available at: https://www.banfield.com/-/media/Project/Banfield/Main/en/general/SOPH-Infographic/PDFs/soph2015_compressed.pdf (accessed 02 October 2022).

Bir, C., Ortez, M., Olynk Widmar, N.J., Wolf, C.A., Hansen, C. *et al.* (2020) Familiarity and use of veterinary services by US resident dog and cat owners. *Animals*, 10(3), E483.

Brown, B.R. (2018) The dimensions of pet-owner loyalty and the relationship with communication, trust, commitment and perceived value. *Veterinary Sciences*, 5(4), 95.

Chandler, M. (2018) Busting pet nutrition myths. *In Focus*. Available at: https://www.veterinary-practice.com/article/busting-pet-nutrition-myths (accessed 16 October 2022).

Cooper, K., Dedehayir, O., Riverola, C., Harrington, S. and Alpert, E. (2022) Exploring consumer perceptions of the value proposition embedded in vegan food products using text analytics. *Sustainability*, 14(4), 2075.

Dodd, S.A., Cave, N.J., Adolphe, J.L., Shoveller, A.K. and Verbrugghe, A. (2019) Plant-based (vegan) diets for pets: A survey of pet owner attitudes and feeding practices. *PLoS ONE*, 14(1), p.e0210806.

Faulkner, B. (2013) The psychology of concordance and compliance. *In Focus*. Available at: https://www.veterinary-practice.com/article/the-psychology-of-concordance-and-compliance (accessed 22 September 2022).

Feather, N.T. (1995) Values, valences and choices: The influence of values on the perceived attractiveness and choice of alternatives. *Journal of Personality and Social Psychology*, 68(6), 1135–1151.

Felsted, K.E. (2012) Building strong relationships among the veterinary team, clients, and patients. *Today's Veterinary Practice*, 2(2), 75–79

Ferrie, S. (2006) A quick guide to ethical theory in healthcare: Solving Ethical dilemmas in nutrition support situations. *Nutrition in Clinical Practice*, 21(2), 113–117.

Food Ethics Council (2022) Understanding food ethics. Available at: https://www.foodethicscouncil.org/learn/food-ethics/ (accessed 13 October 2022).

Fornari, A. (2015) Approaches to ethical decision-making. *The Journal of the Academy of Nutrition and Dietetics,* 115 (1), 119–121.

Gerrard, E. (2015) Owner compliance – educating clients to act on pet care advice. *VN Times*, 15(4), 6–7.

Grand, J.A., Lloyd, J.W., Ilgen, D.R., Abood, S. and Sonea, I.M. (2013) A measure of, and predictors for, veterinarian trust developed with veterinary students in a simulated companion animal practice. *Journal of the American Veterinary Medical Association*, 242, 322–334

Groves, C.N.H., Janke, N., Stroyev, A., Tayce, J.D. and Coe, J.B. (2022) Discussion of cost continues to be uncommon in companion animal veterinary practice. *Journal of the American Veterinary Medical Association*, 260(14), 1844–1852.

Hansen, C. (2021) Stronger client relationships are key to better patient care. *dvm360*, 55 (5), 25–26.

Hassan, A. (2012) The value proposition concept in marketing: How customers perceive the value delivered by firms – a study of customer perspectives on supermarkets in Southampton in the United Kingdom. *International Journal of Marketing Studies*, 4(3), 68–87.

Hauser, W. (2022) How to explain the value and cost of proactive care. *Today's Veterinary Business*, 6(4), 68–72.

Janke, N., Coe, J.B., Bernardo, T.M., Dewey, C.E. and Stone, E.A. (2021) Pet owners' and veterinarians' perceptions of information exchange and clinical decision-making in companion animal practice. *PLoS ONE,* 16(2): e0245632.

Kamleh, M.K., Khosa, D.K., Dewey, C.E., Verbrugghe, A. and Stone, E.A. (2020) Ontario Veterinary College first-year veterinary students' perceptions of companion animal nutrition and their own nutrition: implications for a veterinary nutrition curriculum. *Journal of Veterinary Medical Education*, 48(1), 71–83.

Lewis, D.W. (2017) Myth: We all know what our clients want and need. In: Smith, R.A (ed.) *Proceedings of the Fiftieth Annual Conference, American Association of Bovine Practitioners*. VM Publishing Company, Omaha, Nebraska, pp. 158–161.

Little, G. (2013) Concordance and compliance. *In Focus*. Available at: https://www.veterinary-practice.com/article/concordance-and-compliance (accessed 16 October 2022).

Lue, T.W., Pantenburg, D.P. and Crawford, P.M. (2008) Impact of the owner-pet and client-veterinarian bond on the care that pets receive. *Journal of the American Veterinary Medical Association*, 232(4), 531–540.

MacMartin, C., Wheat, H.C., Coe, J.B. and Adams, C.L. (2018) Conversation analysis of veterinarians' proposals for long-term dietary change in companion animal practice in Ontario, *Canada. Journal of Veterinary Medical Education*, 45(4), 514–533.

McNeill, E. (2018) Food for thought? *Veterinary Focus.* 28(3), 1.

Michel, K.E. (2006) Unconventional diets for dogs and cats. *Veterinary Clinics of North America: Small Animal Practice*, 36(6), 1269–1281.

Michel, K.E., Willoughby, K.N., Abood, S.K., Fascetti, A.J, Fleeman, L.M. *et al.* (2008) Attitudes of pet owners toward pet foods and feeding management of cats and dogs. *Journal of the American Veterinary Medical Association*, 233, 1699–1703.

Milburn, J. (2016) Pet food: Ethical issues. In: Thompson, P. and Kaplan, D. (eds) *Encyclopedia of Food and Agricultural Ethics.* Springer, Dordrecht.

Morgan, C.A. and McDonald, M. (2007) Ethical dilemmas in veterinary medicine. *Veterinary Clinics of North America: Small Animal Practice*, 37, 165–179.

Nolen, S. (2021) Model aims to increase access to veterinary care. American Veterinary Medical Association. Available at: https://avmajournals.avma.org/view/post/news/model-aims-to-increase-access-to-veterinary-care.xml (accessed 30 September 2022).

Payne, A., Frow, P. and Eggert, A. (2017) The customer value proposition: evolution, development, and application in marketing. *The Journal of the Academy of Marketing Science*, 45, 467–489.

Prata, J.C. (2022) Survey of pet owner attitudes on diet choices and feeding practices for their pets in Portugal. *Animals,* 12(20), 2775.

Prendergast, H. (2016) Tips and tricks to rev up your client customer service game. *Today's Veterinary Nurse.* Available at: https://todaysveterinarynurse.com/practice-management/tips-and-tricks-to-rev-up-your-client-service-game/ (accessed 15 September 2022).

Rokeach, M. (1973) *The Nature of Human Values.* Free Press, New York, USA.

Rosenfeld, D.L. (2019) A comparison of dietarian identity profiles between vegetarians and vegans. *Food Quality and Preference,* 72, 40–44.

Rothgerber, H. (2013) A meaty matter. Pet diet and the vegetarian's dilemma. *Appetite,* 68, 76–82.

Tuisku, O.A., Ilves, M.K., Lylykangas, J.K., Surakka, V.V., Ainasoja, M. *et al.* (2018) Emotional responses of clients to veterinarian communication style during a vaccination visit in companion animal practice. *Journal of the American Veterinary Medical Association*, 252(9), 1120–1132.

Tuulik, K., Õunapuu, T., Kuimet, K. and Titov, E. (2016) Rokeach's instrumental and terminal values as descriptors of modern organisation values. *Organizational Communication eJournal.* Available at: https://www.semanticscholar.org/paper/Rokeach%E2%80%99s-Instrumental-and-Terminal-Values-As-of-Tuulik-%C3%95unapuu/f9817aa6ad04cd2c34114ff51bce77bf0031d9a0 (accessed 6 October 2022).

Volk, J.O., Felsted, K.E., Thomas, J.G. and Siren, C.W. (2011) Executive summary of the Bayer veterinary care usage study. *Journal of the American Veterinary Medical Association*, 238(10), 1275–1282.

Zafalon, R.V.A., Risolia, L.W., Vendramini, T.H.A., Ayres Rodrigues, R.B., Pedrinelli, V. *et al.* (2020) Nutritional inadequacies in commercial vegan foods for dogs and cats. *PLoS ONE,* 15(1): e0227046.

Developing an interprofessional nutrition programme: Communication

Tierney Kinnison and Rachel Lumbis

Abstract

Communication skills have been reliably identified as important professional (non-technical) competencies for the success of the veterinary healthcare team (VHCT). A 2016 Best Evidence Medical Education (BEME) guide stated that communication skills were the only competency that was supported by three different categories of evidence (expert frameworks, stakeholder perceptions and empirical research) (Cake *et al.*, 2016). This involved communication with clients and also to a very slightly lesser extent, colleagues. More recently, under the construct of employability, Bell *et al.* (2021) identified communication with clients, communication with colleagues and teamwork as the top three categories ranked by stakeholders when provided with a list. This chapter will examine the communication between professions, primarily considering veterinarians, veterinary nurses (VNs) and technicians, administrators and receptionists, as this has been the focus of research in the veterinary field, as well as bringing in insight from the human medical field. Within this, it will discuss mistakes, errors, blame and the importance of speaking up. The chapter will also explore communication with clients, focusing, in particular, on nutrition conversations. There are multiple reasons, as highlighted in Chapters 3 and 4, why nutrition may not always be top of the discussion list, but this needs to change. Successful communication is key to every step of the nutritional assessment process and is crucial to developing a positive relationship with clients and establishing the VHCT as a vital part of the relationship between pet and caretaker, thus enhancing the human–animal bond (HAB). Clients frequently have a very strong pet bond and caretakers essentially want the best possible care for their pets, but they need to be involved in the dietary decision-making process and receive clear and regular communication to ensure compliance and concordance.

Interprofessional communication

Communication errors

One of the most important potential outcomes of poor communication in a team is that of medical error. It could be claimed that this is an area

DOI: 10.1079/9781800621107.0007

under-researched in the veterinary field, however a few examples provide useful explorations of the situation in veterinary practice. Mellanby and Herrtage (2004) defined an error in their veterinary questionnaire study as 'an erroneous act or omission resulting in a less then optimal or potentially adverse outcome for a patient' and reported that 15/73 recent graduate respondents considered breakdowns in communication between colleagues as a source of their past errors. In a qualitative study involving focus groups, Oxtoby *et al.* (2015) related communication to poor leadership and teamwork and identified several aspects of communication between colleagues as causes of error, including poor transfer of information at handovers, lack of speaking up, lack of asking for help and informal processes which relied on assumptions rather than protocols. Kinnison *et al.* (2015) took a slightly wider view of error, incorporating inputs or omitted actions with potential adverse outcomes for patients, clients or the practice, and reported 40 instances of errors observed during fieldwork. Communication errors were the largest group of errors and pertained to mistakes in records, procedures, missing face-to-face communication and mistakes as part of face-to-face communication. Information here was split into missing or incorrect (mistake). Information may be missing, i.e., withheld, for a variety of reasons according to the general interprofessional literature, including cognitive blindness (where one profession filters out information which would have been useful to another profession due to lack of understanding), confidentiality, limited time and stress (Barr *et al.*, 2005).

The majority of the communication errors reported by Kinnison *et al.* (2015) involved veterinary surgeons and receptionists, with interviews of these groups highlighting a tension between the veterinary surgeon's desire for individual autonomy in action and the receptionist's wishes for standard procedures to follow, rather than remembering individual preferences.

Medical error has been more closely researched in human healthcare. One example (Lingard *et al.*, 2004) which nicely considers broad types of communication errors in operating rooms suggests that there are:

- **Occasion failures**: problems in the situation or context of the communication event. For example, a question being asked which is too late to be of assistance.
- **Content failures**: insufficient or inaccurate information communicated. For example, inaccurate information regarding the patient's treatment so far.
- **Audience failures**: gaps in the composition of the group involved. For example, discussions taking place when a key member of the team is missing, and often requiring further discussion upon their return.
- **Purpose failures**: the purpose of the communication is unclear, not achieved, or inappropriate. For example, questions are discussed, but an answer or plan is not formed.

As many of these examples show, mistakes can and should largely be considered as system errors rather than errors of an individual. While it is true that, on occasion, an individual will make a mistake due to a lack of, for example, cognitive awareness of the situation, it is perhaps more common for mistakes to happen for a variety of contributing reasons attributed to the system, rather than just one individual. Therefore, while striving for a 'just culture' whereby an individual should face repercussions for failure to learn and behave appropriately despite guidance (Wachter and Pronovost, 2009), it is largely unhelpful to look for someone to blame. Despite this, blame is an identified feature of the work by Kinnison *et al.* (2015) whereby examples were seen of the clinical professions blaming receptionists, though it is noted that examples were also seen of clinical professions sharing the blame for a mistake. Understanding the demands on each other is therefore important, especially for receptionists who are constantly dealing with clients face to face, on the phone and via email, as well as often being the central link in communication between clients and clinical staff, despite having unstandardised training and understandably a lack of knowledge regarding medical issues. This aligns with the concept of 'situational awareness' which has been described as including individual factors (such as comprehension of the situation), team factors (including shared awareness, shared mental models and shared projection regarding the future), in addition to representation of surroundings (e.g., displays), team communication and teamwork (e.g., trust and respect) (Graafland *et al.*, 2015).

A useful way to think about systems errors is James Reason's (2000) 'Swiss cheese' model. Consider several slices of Swiss cheese (the type with holes) all lined up. Sometimes a hole in one slice will be covered by cheese from another slice. Sometimes though, the holes will line up, and something could pass right through. This is the error – sometimes it will be stopped, by an individual speaking up, or by a good, standardised procedure, for example. Sometimes it will get through and the error will happen. One person may be at the end of the line, but to learn from our mistakes, we must look more closely than just at this one individual.

While the types of errors mentioned so far lend themselves to consideration of mistakes in surgery, for example, lessons can be taken for consideration of mistakes and errors in nutritional practice. This could include missing information in handovers from veterinary healthcare team (VHCT) members admitting a patient and those undertaking its immediate care, failure to create a suitable plan for the nutritional care of a patient, and decisions about nutritional plans being made without key members of the team being present.

Speak up or salute and stay mute?

A pertinent aspect of team communication mentioned already a couple of times in this chapter is speaking up, the opposite of the catchy term 'salute and stay mute', coined by Patterson *et al.* (2001). This can relate to speaking up in the moment, to usually address a safety concern to a patient, or speaking up after an event to ensure it is recorded and lessons can be learned. Most of the research applies to the former definition. Several studies in human healthcare have investigated the occurrence of speaking up, and the challenges with doing so. In one study within a radiology department of a single US institution, 50% of respondents spoke up about safety concerns all the time, meaning another 50% spoke up less than all the time, ranging from most of the time to never (Siewert *et al.*, 2018). In an Australian university hospital, three departments (surgery, anaesthesiology and intensive care medicine and internal medicine) took part in a survey which researched different aspects of speaking up, and, for example, 16.4% of 859 respondents reported that they remained silent when they had information that might have prevented a safety incident in their unit at least once within the last four weeks (Schwappach *et al.*, 2018). This study reported no differences between physicians' and nurses' behaviour in all aspects of speaking up. These two examples highlight the prevalence of not speaking up, and while similar research has not been conducted in the veterinary field, it can be assumed that due to similarities in the professional make-up of the teams and the type of work undertaken, veterinary surgeons, VNs, receptionists and other groups will also experience this lack of speaking up. It is important therefore to unpack this complicated decision and aim to address barriers to speaking up.

Kobayashi *et al.* (2006) conducted a questionnaire study with residents in the US and Japan and concluded that whether a resident would challenge their superior was related to their relationship with the individual, and their perception of the response from the superior staff member. Opinions on some aspects regarding the workplace differed between the two countries' responses, including for example 'Doctors who encourage suggestions from other junior members are weak leaders', whereby 97.1% of US respondents did not find this consistent with their beliefs compared to 77.6% of Japanese respondents. However, the threshold for challenge was not different, suggesting challenges of professional and organisational culture are likely to be greater than challenges of national culture. In a literature review, Okuyama *et al.* (2014) researched speaking up behaviour and the links between speaking up and patient safety. In total, 27 articles were included which enabled the identification of factors affecting speaking up, as summarised below:

- the motivation to speak up, such as the perceived risk for patients
- contextual factors, such as administrative support, relationship between team members, attitude of leaders/superiors
- individual factors, such as job satisfaction, confidence based on experience, communication skills
- the perceived efficacy of speaking up, such as lack of impact and personal control
- the perceived safety of speaking up, such as fear for the responses of others and conflict and concerns over appearing incompetent
- tactics and targets, such as showing positive intent.

In the radiology study previously mentioned, high reporting threshold, which incorporates the conviction that you are right, was the most frequent barrier for speaking up overall, and for nursing and administration staff, while residents/fellows most frequently reported challenging authority as a barrier (Siewert *et al.*, 2018).

Specific questionnaires have been designed to measure aspects of speaking up among medical staff. One recent example by Aline *et al.* (2021) discusses principal component analysis (which allows questionnaire items receiving similar rankings from respondents to be grouped together into scales), and the identification of a structure of three speaking-up behaviour-related scales (frequency of perceived concerns, withholding voice and speaking up), in addition to three scales of 'speak-up climate' (psychological safety, encouraging environment and resignation).

It is clear from these examples that individual veterinary practices which develop their own cultures, as well as the professions as a whole, need to advance a culture whereby speaking up is encouraged, negative ramifications are not experienced, and hierarchies are flattened.

In a veterinary practice it is therefore important that all members of the VHCT feel empowered to speak up regarding potential nutritional issues. Such issues may include veterinarians' failure to incorporate nutritional assessments into their consultations (if this has been agreed as standard practice by the practice team), inaccurate or incomplete information transfer between staff regarding a patient's nutritional care, nutritional plans with which they disagree or if personal nutritional expertise is not being utilised.

Learning from mistakes

In addition to attempting to reduce errors in real time, it is important to encourage a team's ability to learn from mistakes and near misses. Initially this requires teams to be comfortable in reporting errors and near misses, which is likely to have similar barriers to speaking up during an incident. Subsequently, it also requires the team to be able to hold meetings which foster a no-blame culture and promote learning. The Veterinary Defence Society (VDS) has several resources on its tool 'VetSafe' (VDS, 2021) which aims to help veterinary practices understand why mistakes happened, develop solutions to improve practice, and support the team members involved in mistakes, known as second victims. One resource outlines a suggested format for mortality and morbidity meetings. This includes aspects of root cause analysis, a structured approach to investigate errors without focusing on blame. While critiques of the term 'root cause analysis' suggest there is not usually one single root cause, and that the purpose of such a meeting is not to find the cause per se, but to identify ways forwards from the error event (Taylor-Adams and Vincent, n.d.), it is still a useful term to remember when conducting such meetings. The structure of such a meeting is likely to involve detailed consideration of the 'contributory factors' to a 'care delivery problem' (the error), and in the veterinary field these have been summarised by VDS as potentially including:

- patient factors
- owner factors
- individual (staff) factors
- task factors
- team factors
- communication factors
- education and training factors
- equipment and resources factors
- working conditions factors
- organisational and strategic factors.

Such meetings should be interprofessional and representative of the teams involved, and those groups who could contribute to the discussion, no matter their profession or status. While such meetings are likely to be time consuming, and at times uncomfortable, they are vital to change our mistakes, errors and near-misses into learning opportunities for the benefit of our patients, clients, team and ourselves.

Communication between the VHCT and clients

While communication with colleagues is seen as an important skill for veterinarians, when communication is considered in the undergraduate education of this group, it almost universally relates to communication with clients (Mossop *et al.*, 2015) and rarely, if ever, to communication with colleagues. Communication with clients is a frequent source of research regarding veterinary surgeons, with almost 800 results from the search 'veterinary communication client' in Pubmed in 2022, with a clear increase in publications in 2006 and again in 2016, culminating in 114 publications in 2021 alone.

Models of communication

A frequently referenced model of client communication for veterinary surgeons is the Calgary-Cambridge Observation Guide. As this model was designed in human medicine for doctors and their patients, modifications have been required for the veterinary field, and are described in the first citing of the model in the *Journal of Veterinary Medical Education* (Adams and Ladner, 2004). In this guide, the overall tasks of a consultation are explored: '(1) initiating the appointment, (2) gathering information, (3) developing a relationship, (4) explaining and planning, and (5) closing the session' (p. 139). It is stated that while these tasks mostly occur in the sequence presented, relationship development occurs throughout. It was not until 2021 that a specific framework for consultations by VNs with their clients was published (Macdonald *et al.*, 2021). This framework, the Veterinary Nurse–Client Communication Matrix (VNCCM), identifies the components of communication between VN and client and outlines the skills and approaches that can be used to achieve these components. It is suggested to have an innovative approach to communication, with a focus on aspects such as motivational interviewing, shared decision-making, achieving informed consent and reflection. Such models offer a helpful guide in ensuring effective communication with clients and all members of the VHCT are encouraged to access and revisit these on a regular basis and utilise them in training.

Enhancing communication

Effective communication is fundamental to establishing a reliable and trustful relationship between the VHCT and pet caretakers. The selection of appropriate language, style of communication, information exchange process, decision-making support and empowerment of all members of the VHCT to engage in appropriate conversations can impact many outcomes of veterinary care. These include patient care, caretakers' understanding of pet health and welfare (Janke *et al.*, 2021), client satisfaction (Coe *et al.*, 2010), veterinarian satisfaction (Shaw *et al.*, 2012) and information recall (Latham and Morris, 2007), caretaker adherence (Kanji *et al.*, 2012) and consultation efficiency and accuracy (Dysart *et al.*, 2011). This is particularly pertinent when discussing nutrition and emotive topics such as weight management and unconventional feeding, which can be challenging and uncomfortable for pet caretakers and the VHCT. Breakdowns in communication and information exchange can have a detrimental impact on the client–VHCT relationship, causing caretakers to question the motivations of the VHCT (Janke *et al.*, 2021).

Tips to enhance VHCT–client communication include:

- VHCT demonstration of:
  ○ reliability and competence (Pun, 2020)
  ○ kindness, compassion and empathy in communication (Küper and Merle, 2019)
  ○ interest in the treatment and welfare of animals (Rujoiu and Rujoju, 2016) and ability to forge a personal connection with the caretaker and their pet (Ward, 2022a)
  ○ effective non-verbal communication, including the maintenance of good eye contact (Abood and Verton-Shaw, 2021)
  ○ respect for caretakers' individuality (Küper and Merle, 2019) and their beliefs and viewpoint (Cline *et al.*, 2021).
  ○ patience and confidence (Küper and Merle, 2019)
  ○ non-judgemental attitude (Küper and Merle, 2019)

     o   active listening skills, allowing the conversation to progress naturally, rather than simply instructing and recording dictation (Ward, 2022a)

     o   willingness to share their own (nutrition-related) personal experiences (Pun, 2020).

- Providing sufficient time to engage in conversation (Pun, 2020).
- Use of relatively simple language and the avoidance of jargon (Nickels and Feeley, 2018).
- Careful consideration of the choice of words used when gathering a nutritional history. For example, pet caretakers may be more likely to admit to giving their pet a food 'reward' or 'training aid' than a 'treat'. Similarly, enquiring about the foods a caretaker 'shares with their pet' may elicit a more comprehensive and accurate response than asking about any 'table scraps' or 'leftovers' being fed. More information is provided on this later in the chapter.
- Using an appropriate pace of verbal communication that accommodates assimilation of information (Küper and Merle, 2019).
- Informing clients of all possible options for the care and treatment of their pet, regardless of cost (Pun, 2020). This reduces clients' concerns over the VHCT's financial motivations behind the recommendations being made (Janke *et al.*, 2021).
- Providing the opportunity for caretakers to ask questions without being made to feel foolish or rushed (Küper and Merle, 2019; Pun, 2020).
- Repeating key information (Küper and Merle, 2019).
- Signposting to credible further information (Pun, 2020).

Feeding nutrition into conversations

Every client visit is an opportunity to discuss the importance of good pet nutrition and body weight. As highlighted in Chapter 8, it is important for each veterinary practice to define its own philosophy on nutrition and to train and leverage all members of the VHCT to maximise all available opportunities to broach the topic of nutrition. Communication must be effective and successful at every step from nutritional assessment and recommendations, through to follow-up and reassessment. It should be an iterative, rather than a linear, process that considers factors relating to the animal and its diet, environment and caretaker (Fig. 7.1) and evaluates the changing nutritional requirements of a pet throughout its life and according to the presence of disease and any comorbidities.

    Routine nutrition conversations with caretakers can help to establish the VHCT as the experts on their pet's nutrition and the primary source of information. Normalising communication regarding a pet's diet, weight status and the health risks associated with obesity can also help to support greater caretaker awareness and the establishment of a weight management partnership

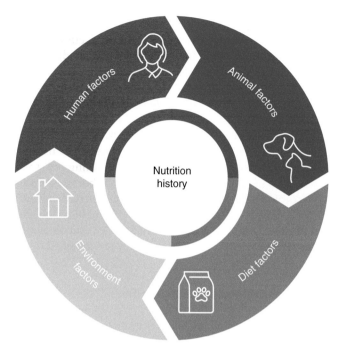

Fig. 7.1. Components of a comprehensive nutritional history. Reprinted with permission from the *2021 AAHA Nutrition and Weight Management Guidelines for Dogs and Cats*. Copyright © 2022 American Animal Hospital Association (aaha.org).

between client and the VHCT (Wainwright *et al.*, 2022). As outlined by Cline *et al.* (2021, p. 163), three aspects of communication are involved in a nutrition conversation:

1. Content: the medical or scientific knowledge that informs a complete and balanced nutrition recommendation.

2. Process: the approach used to engage a client in discussion about their pet's nutrition.

3. Perception: how the client thinks and feels about pet nutrition, including their assumptions, beliefs, goals, thought processes and decision-making.

As discussed in Chapter 6, the development of trust, empathy and rapport is crucial in the relationship between clients and the VHCT and is fundamental to effective communication about nutrition and dietary choice (Abood and Verton-Shaw, 2021). It can enhance the quality of a nutritional history and promote the prescription of a more comprehensive nutritional recommendation. Inviting the caretaker to enter into a nutrition conversation and seeking their permission to proceed (Ward, 2022b) can gauge their receptivity to discuss nutrition and shows respect (Cline *et al.*, 2021). For example: 'Based on my assessment of Lewis today, I feel that we could make some small dietary changes to help improve his health. I have some ideas regarding food and snacks. Would you be interested in discussing this today?'

It is also vital to understand the pet caretaker's perspective, beliefs and goals, alongside the recognition and management of your own nutrition-related biases and perceptions (Cline *et al.*, 2021). Obtaining a nutritional history prior to the pet's arrival can help to increase the accuracy of information provision and reduce any feelings of pet caretaker judgement or pressure. On arrival at the practice, appropriate questioning, using a combination of open and closed questions, can then be used to obtain a narrative nutritional history (Ward, 2022a), with equal consideration of animal-, diet-, environment-, and human-related factors (Table 7.1). As outlined in Chapter 8, utilising the skills of VNs to collect information prior to consultation with a veterinarian and to provide other specific VN-led services can have several benefits. These include the provision of more time and cost-effective practice and enabling veterinarians to focus on the completion of tasks only they are qualified to complete.

Communicating a nutritional recommendation

The veterinary decision-making process is acknowledged to be one of the most complex aspects of the interaction between veterinarian, client and patient (Janke *et al.*, 2021). The approach to communication taken by the VHCT can impact caretakers' involvement in this process and their engagement and ultimate satisfaction (Janke *et al.*, 2021; Ito *et al.*, 2022). When both a VN and veterinarian communicate with clients, Janke *et al.* (2022) found that caretakers are more involved in decision-making regarding their pet's healthcare. Furthermore, VNs' communication significantly enhanced client engagement in decision-making when working collaboratively with the veterinarian. It is thus important to build strong partnerships in veterinary decision processes (Küper and Merle, 2019) and reduce transactional interactions between veterinary practices and clients. As Janke *et al.* (2021) reported, pet caretakers expect support in making informed decisions and require the VHCT to understand their current knowledge, be able to tailor information accordingly and educate them about their opinions (Fig. 7.2). But when the professional advice and information provided contradicts a caretaker's beliefs, values or behaviour, the resultant discomfort and conflict can result in cognitive dissonance whereby information is selectively processed, and misaligned information is disregarded.

To be successful, communication of a nutritional recommendation needs to be comprehensible and unambiguous; if a healthcare recommendation makes sense and is explained well, with a clear rationale, it can be up to seven times more likely to be accepted and followed (Kanji *et al.*, 2012). On average, the compliance rate with veterinary medicine is 15–60%, but less than 20% of caretakers follow pet feeding instructions (AAHA, 2003, 2009; Davies, 2012). A significant compliance gap is evident between the nutritional recommendations that veterinarians believe are being implemented and those that

Table 7.1. Examples of open and closed questions used in nutrition-related conversations and history-taking. Adapted with permission from the *2021 AAHA Nutrition and Weight Management Guidelines for Dogs and Cats* (aaha.org).

	Open questions	Closed questions
Animal factors	• Explain how 'Buster' has been since his last visit, including any changes or concerns you may have.	• Has Buster experienced any changes in his food intake or behaviour/health? For example, – amount eaten – chewing – swallowing – vomiting – regurgitation – diarrhoea – flatulence – constipation?
Diet factors	• Explain what factors influence your choice of pet food. • Imagine that I am going to be looking after Buster. What would I need to know in relation to his diet and feeding requirements? • Describe any additional food that Buster receives in addition to his canned food/kibble. This would include food rewards, chew toys, supplements, food used to administer medication and any table food.	• Has Buster's food intake changed recently? • How much and how frequently do you feed Buster each day? • Where and how do you usually store Buster's food? • What food do you like to share with Buster?
Environment factors	• Tell me how Buster gets on with everyone in the household, including people and other pets. • Explain which members of the household have responsibility for feeding Buster, including his meals and other food sources such as rewards or snacks. • Imagine that I am going to be looking after Buster. What would I need to know in relation to his usual daily routine, activities and exercise?	• Does Buster spend most of his time indoors or outdoors? • Are there any environmental stressors at home (e.g. recent changes in the home or uncontrollable outdoor stimuli)? • What favourite activities do you like to participate in with Buster? • Where do you usually feed Buster?
Human factors	• What is most important when you consider Buster's diet? • What questions or concerns do you have regarding Buster's diet? • Tell me about what you have already read/learnt regarding pet nutrition.	• Besides what we have discussed already, is there any additional information that you would find helpful?

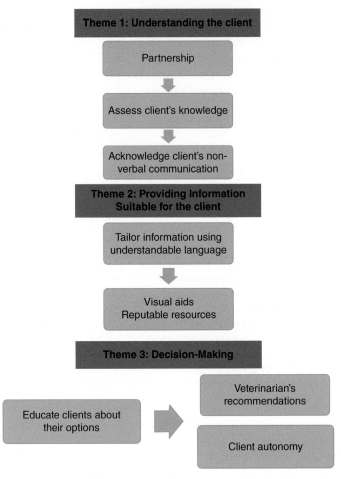

Fig. 7.2. A concept map of the themes and subthemes related to information exchange and decision-making expectations that emerged from pet owner focus groups. Reprinted Janke *et al.* (2021), distributed under the terms of Creative Commons Attribution 4.0 International Public License and with permission from journals.plos.org.

are executed by pet owners (AAHA, 2003; Bergler *et al.*, 2016). The higher the pet–caretaker and vet–client bond, the higher the level of care expected, meaning an increased likelihood of recommendations being followed, regardless of cost (Lue *et al.*, 2008). Successful communication also requires consistency and reinforcement from all members of the VHCT (Ward, 2022c). Although often only one member of the VHCT is in consultation with a client at a time, Russell *et al.* (2022) advocate that, when viewed in its entirety, communication is a collective competence, requiring the consideration of systems and teams rather than individuals. The importance of this is supported by the finding in their research of cases of alleged professional negligence whereby problems in communication were a factor in 80% of cases. Churchill and Ward (2016) also advocate for a team approach to nutritional counselling, observing that a consistent and unified approach from the VHCT is needed, while still acknowledging the importance of individuality in terms of communication approaches between professionals and the diverse needs of different clients. This ensures that all members of the team are aware of the history of a patient and the plan, and this can be achieved through appropriately written patient notes as well as verbal communication.

Cline *et al.* (2021) provide a general framework for communicating a nutrition recommendation (Fig. 7.3). Further tips for successful communication are provided below and in the subsequent section.

- Educate about the benefits and risks of each nutrition option (Cline *et al.*, 2021).
- Ensure that the recommendation aligns with the caretaker's own goals and beliefs (Cline *et al.*, 2021) and highlights how it will benefit the health and welfare of the pet.
- Ask the caretaker to repeat back their interpretation of their pet's nutritional recommendation to identify any potential misunderstanding or miscommunication.
- Provide a verbal and written recap of the main points that have been discussed, thus reinforcing the advice given. Provided sufficient notes are made on the patient's record, the latter could be provided by another member of the VHCT, not just a veterinarian or veterinary nurse.

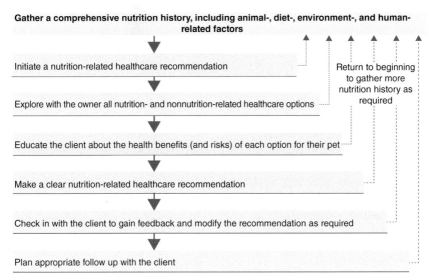

Fig. 7.3. A general framework for communicating a nutrition-related healthcare recommendation. Reprinted with permission from the *2021 AAHA Nutrition and Weight Management Guidelines for Dogs and Cats.* Copyright © 2022 American Animal Hospital Association (aaha.org).

- Use closed questioning to ensure that the caretaker is happy, they have the resources and information they need, and to ensure that their expectations for the consultation have been met.
- Ensure the availability and use of a range of resources and educational materials to help communicate the nutritional recommendation (Abood and Verton-Shaw, 2021), such as:
  - a nutrition history form, including an overview of the four factors that form a nutrition history (Fig. 7.1)
  - body condition and muscle condition scores (BCS and MCS), while noting that non-sequential BCS images have been identified as a potentially useful resource for promoting a more considered opinion of canine weight status by caretakers (Wainwright *et al.*, 2022)
  - faecal score charts
  - calorie needs for healthy adult dogs and cats
  - nutrition brochures and leaflets, including frequently-asked questions
  - an 'information prescription' containing veterinary recommended online nutrition resources
  - appointment cards and details of how to contact the VHCT and/or the practice's nutrition champion.

Discussing controversial topics

Potentially controversial topics include the feeding of unconventional diets, such as raw and meat-based diets, grain-free, vegan/vegetarian and insect-based, as well as discussions surrounding weight management. The motivations for feeding alternative diets, including those that are home-made, include:

- a requirement as part of a diet elimination trial or due to food sensitivities
- therapeutic diets are either unavailable or unacceptable, particularly if pets have comorbidities
- caretakers' desire to:
  - make their pet's meals
  - utilise more environmentally friendly and sustainable ingredients
  - avoid feeding carbohydrates, grains, gluten and other ingredients or nutrients perceived as being undesirable
  - feed a more 'natural' diet for perceived improved coat condition, dental health and stool quality
- appeal of whole or organic foods and vegetarian or vegan diets
- concerns about additives, preservatives or ingredients used in commercial pet foods
- reasons relating to animal ethics (Newton *et al.*, 2019).

Yet most homemade diets are not complete or balanced and risks include nutritional deficiencies and excesses (Niza *et al.*, 2003; Verbrugghe *et al.*, 2011; Heinze *et al.*, 2012; Larsen *et al.*, 2012; Stockman *et al.*, 2013; Sontas *et al.*,

2014; Wilson *et al.*, 2019). The safety and suitability of vegan and raw food diets is also questionable, with a substantial body of literature available on the potential risks of raw feeding to pets, caretakers and the wider public (Joffe and Schlesinger, 2002; Stiver *et al.*, 2003; Weese *et al.*, 2005; Strohmeyer *et al.*, 2006; Schotte *et al.*, 2007; Yin, 2007; Finley *et al.*, 2008; Behravesh *et al.*, 2010; Buchanan *et al.*, 2011; Freeman *et al.*, 2013; Nemser *et al.*, 2014; Nilsson, 2015; van Bree *et al.*, 2018; Groat *et al.*, 2022). Nevertheless, people are not always willing to change their minds, even when informed about the dangers and limitations of their decisions and faced with evidence-based information. Perceived effectiveness of guidance is an important indicator of caretakers' nutrition behaviours for their pets (Kamleh *et al.*, 2020). However, knowledge and awareness, alone, is insufficient to produce or change behaviour unless accompanied by a change in attitudes and the provision of support.

Holding a difficult conversation about an uncomfortable subject requires consideration of how the topic is raised, the words used and the tone in which they are spoken (Mulrooney, 2019, p. 349). Motivational interviewing and the '5 As' model are used in human medicine to promote patient behaviour change, including smoking cessation, dietary change, and reduction in alcohol consumption and weight. Using a linear and sequential format, healthcare practitioners are encouraged to 'Ask' (e.g., for permission to discuss diet and weight), and then 'Assess' (e.g., nutritional assessment), 'Advise' (e.g., inform about the risks associated with obesity), 'Agree' (e.g., set goals and expectations) and 'Assist' or 'Arrange' (e.g., discuss options, provide support or expert referral). Preliminary findings of an international study by Hodgkiss *et al.* (2020) indicated caretakers' preference for a modified 5A framework during pet weight management consultations. This patient-centred approach involves 'Asking' before entering a cyclical process, through which the remaining four As are considered.

In Churchill and Ward's (2016) exploration of communicating with pet owners about obesity, it is observed that pet owners will go through different stages in their readiness for behavioural change regarding addressing obesity. This descriptive report helpfully presents detailed ideas regarding ways to discuss obesity during these different stages, moving from showing concern when the client is not yet ready to change, to finding out more about the pet's context through open-ended questions and sharing relevant resources, to developing individual weight loss plans, including refinements and acceptance of setbacks. It is possible that the use of a tool which naturally avoids judgement, such as a quality-of-life questionnaire, may be beneficial, and may also aid alignment of stakeholder goals (Hanford and Linder, 2021).

When entering a potentially contentious conversation or managing cognitive dissonance, it is important to:

- Emphasise that you are in partnership with the caretaker and, ultimately, both want the same goal of optimising their pet's health, welfare, wellbeing, quality of life and longevity, while ensuring that the diet fed is safe for all household members (humans and animals). Highlighting common ground, while also promoting a safe and relaxed environment, can help improve receptivity to new information (Chandler, 2018).

- Be aware of own judgements and biases, together with consideration of body language, so these do not undermine the relationship and trust between client and VHCT. In human medicine, the bias and prejudice against obese people results in poorer provision of healthcare (Fitch and Bays, 2022). In veterinary medicine, a small-scale survey by Sutherland *et al.* (2022) identified the presence of weight bias, with an unconscious preference by veterinary professionals for thin people. Findings by Pearl *et al.* (2020) have also revealed:
    - o veterinarians and veterinary students feel more blame, frustration and disgust towards obese dogs and obese owners compared to lean dogs and lean owners
    - o obese owners of overweight dogs are perceived as causing their dog's obesity, while lean owners are thought to be responsible for their dogs being lean
    - o the use of stigmatising language is common.
- Gather a comprehensive nutrition history.
- Enquire what the client's reasons are behind their diet selection and feeding behaviours in a non-threatening manner (Ward, 2022a), while recognising that they have likely acted in good faith. Focus on understanding their concerns, expectations and goals to ensure alignment when making a nutritional recommendation.
- Specifically ask what the caretaker's concerns are and listen to and validate these before discussing and suggesting any changes.
- Focus on presenting and repeating facts and stress any misguided beliefs to reinforce these using a non-antagonistic approach (Chandler, 2018). Correct, evidence-based information should be provided together with an explanation of why the misconception is wrong (however, overwhelming pet caretakers with too much detail can prevent a proper conversation).
- Acknowledge that the caretaker is feeding a diet they believe to be most appropriate for, and in the best interests of, their pet while realising this is not an endorsement or agreement with their decision making.
- Inform about the potential risks and benefits of the diet choice.
- Highlight any good feeding practice and behaviours demonstrated by the caretaker.
- Focus on the pet's nutritional requirements and what is best for its health and wellbeing. Along with consideration of the caretaker's beliefs, preferences and circumstances (e.g., budget and consideration of all human and non-human household members), this should form the basis of an individualised nutritional recommendation. When discussing a pet's diet

in the context of its health during a wellness appointment, a primary care veterinarian may be most persuasive to the caretaker for changing their pet's diet (Alvarez and Schultz, 2021).

- Recognise that the way you frame a nutritional recommendation to a pet caretaker is likely to impact on their willingness to accept and follow it (Mulrooney, 2019).
- Consider appropriate use of language and avoid terms that could be perceived as derogatory, particularly when discussing weight. These include plump, fat, obese, chubby and heavy for describing a high body condition score and scrawny, sleek and skinny for describing a low BCS (Hodgkiss *et al.*, 2020). Focus the conversation on quality of life, disease reduction and the promotion of health, wellbeing and longevity (Cline *et al.*, 2021), using resources such as BCS to support recommendations (Abood and Verton-Shaw, 2021).
- Recognise that different clients require different approaches to communication (e.g. direct versus indirect and scientific versus emotional). Some may also prefer to discuss the nutritional recommendation with a non-veterinarian.
- Accept that there will always be clients who question the VHCT's motivations behind the nutritional recommendations being made. Despite best efforts, not all will be convinced to alter the feeding management of their pet, even when the consequences of not doing so are detrimental to the pet's health and wellbeing. Be your patients' nutritional advocate – consider any potential compromises to improve their diet and consult with a Board-Certified Veterinary Nutritionist or a European Board of Veterinary Specialisation (EBVS) Specialist in Veterinary and Comparative Nutrition, if required (further information in Chapter 3).
- Include a comprehensive record of the nutritional assessment, including nutritional history, and recommendation in the pet's medical record.

Along with communication and information provision, the behaviour and attitude of caretakers heavily influences their feeding behaviours and adherence to nutritional recommendations (Kamleh *et al.*, 2020). Caretakers have ultimate responsibility for caring for and determining the quality of life of their pet, thus highlighting the importance of behaviour change and placing it at the heart of veterinary practice (Bard *et al.*, 2017). It is important to ensure that all members of the VHCT are aware of the existing research in this area and have been trained appropriately and have the necessary confidence and competence to conduct such conversations. Providing training in communication skills and motivational interviewing techniques can enable the VHCT to better assess a client's readiness to change, and thus their likelihood of compliance with nutritional recommendations, as well as supporting them in overcoming resistance to changing attitudes and behaviours (Abood and Verton-Shaw, 2021).

The challenges of nutrition conversations

As outlined in Chapter 3, many household animals are considered irreplaceable family members (Ito *et al.*, 2022). For many caretakers, their affection or love for their pets is most pronounced through the provision of food, with over half giving equal or more priority to buying healthy food for their pets compared to themselves (Schleicher *et al.*, 2019). As recognised by Mulrooney (2019, p. 349), 'Eating is about far more than nutrition or calories; it is about love, nurturing and acceptance.' The HAB and relationship between pet and caretaker is an important factor in pet food purchase behaviour (Schleicher *et al.*, 2019) and so questioning a caretaker's pet dietary decision making can be incorrectly perceived as inferring a lack of care or love for the pet. Many caretakers will select the diet they believe to be most appropriate for their pet and this may reflect their own cultural beliefs, ideologies and dietary preferences. Advertising can prove persuasive, particularly when it targets the emotional attachment between caretaker and pet, and the 'humanisation' of pet food and ascribing of human predilections to companion animals is a significant trend influencing the pet food industry (Fig. 7.4). However, animals' nutritional requirements are dissimilar, and the ingredients and quantity of food consumed by humans may not necessarily be safe or appropriate for consumption by companion animals (Clemens, 2014). Other factors influencing caretakers' pet food selection and purchase are outlined in Chapter 3.

Pet feeding habits and diet choice are highly emotive and sensitive topics for many caretakers, and potentially also controversial, making nutrition conversations challenging. As identified in Chapter 4, this is one of the many

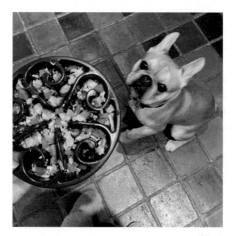

Fig. 7.4. Clients' pet food philosophies often closely follow their personal food choices. Some caretakers will ascribe their own human predilections to their pets on a regular basis, while others do so on occasions, such as illustrated here at Christmas. Photograph: author.

reasons that nutrition is seldom and infrequently discussed with clients at veterinary visits. Yet caretakers want, and need, valid, reliable and evidence-based information on optimal pet nutrition and feeding management. Normalising nutrition conversations and emphasising nutrition's impact on a pet's health and wellbeing is crucial and can help to preserve the bond between pets and caretakers, making it an essential responsibility of the VHCT. As identified by Alvarez *et al.* (2022), nutrition conversations with clients have been perceived by veterinarians as positive interactions, so finding ways to overcome barriers to starting these conversations is key.

Clients who take a more proactive role in their pet's health are increasingly aware of correct nutrition as a key factor in optimising animal health, wellbeing, performance and quality of life. However, as outlined in Chapter 3, there is a growing distrust in veterinary advice and influence of cognitive bias in decision-making. Not all pet caretakers consider the VHCT to be their primary and trusted source of nutritional information and may instead refer to, and favour, information that reinforces their own views and beliefs. This can be biased, inaccurate and outdated, leading to misinformation, misperceptions and misunderstanding. It is, therefore, crucial for the VHCT to establish an emotional connection, broach the topic of nutrition and hold open and emotionally neutral conversations about pet feeding habits and diet choice.

In summary

The ability to effectively communicate, within and between veterinary teams and with clients, is a core, collective competence for veterinary professionals and is fundamental to high quality veterinary care, client satisfaction and increased client compliance with veterinary recommendations. Communication failure can quickly lead to misunderstandings or treatment errors and give cause for complaint and litigation, ultimately influencing the success of a veterinary practice. With increased importance being placed on the HAB and the associated public demand for extended services and high quality care in veterinary medicine, the ability to communicate in a kind, respectful and informative manner is a key requirement and expectation of pet caretakers when interacting with the VHCT. Simply communicating the importance of nutrition and appropriate dietary choice to pet caretakers and the VHCT does not always change behaviour; information provision, together with consistent and long-term support is needed to alter and maintain new behaviours. A purposeful and inclusive approach to nutrition education can help to promote nutrition conversations but this is reliant on contribution and buy-in from the entire veterinary team, ideally including one or more 'nutritional champions'.

References

AAHA (American Animal Hospital Association) (2003) *The Path to High-Quality Care: Practical Tips for Improving Compliance.* AAHA Press, Lakewood, Colorado.

AAHA (American Animal Hospital Association) (2009) *Compliance: Taking Quality Care to the Next Level: A Report of the 2009 AAHA Compliance Follow-up Study.* AAHA Press, Lakewood, Colorado.

Abood, S.K. and Verton-Shaw, S. (2021) Talking about dog and cat nutrition with clients. *Veterinary Clinics of North America: Small Animal Practice,* 51 (3), 517–528.

Adams, C. L. and Ladner, L. (2004) Implementing a simulated client program: Bridging the gap between theory and practice. *Journal of Veterinary Medical Education,* 31(2), 138–145.

Aline, R., Pfeiffer, Y. and Schwappach, D.D.L. (2021) Development and psychometric evaluation of the Speaking Up About Patient Safety Questionnaire. *Journal of Patient Safety,* 17(7), e599–e606.

Alvarez, E.E. and Schultz, K.K. (2021) Effect of personal, food manufacturer, and pet health statements made by a veterinarian during a pet wellness appointment on a dog or cat owner's decision to consider changing their pet's diet. *Journal of the American Veterinary Medical Association,* 259(6), 644–650.

Alvarez, E.E., Schultz, K.K., Floerchinger, A.M. and Hull, J.L. (2022) Small animal general practitioners discuss nutrition infrequently despite assertion of indication, citing barriers. *Journal of the American Veterinary Medical Association,* 260(13), 1704–1710.

Bard, A.M., Main, D.C.J., Haase, A.M., Whay, H.R., Roe, E.J. *et al.* (2017) The future of veterinary communication: Partnership or persuasion? A qualitative investigation of veterinary communication in the pursuit of client behaviour change. *PLoS ONE,* 12(3), e0171380.

Barr, H., Koppel, I., Reeves, S., Hammick, M. and Freeth, D. (2005) *Effective Interprofessional Education: Argument, Assumption and Evidence,* Blackwell Publishing Ltd, Oxford, UK.

Behravesh, C.B., Ferraro, A., Deasy, M., Dato, V., Moll, M. *et al.* (2010) Human *Salmonella* infections linked to contaminated dry dog and cat food, 2006–2008. *Pediatrics,* 126, 477–483.

Bell, M.A., Cake, M. and Mansfield, C.F. (2021) International multi-stakeholder consensus for the capabilities most important to employability in the veterinary profession. *Veterinary Record,* 188(5), e20.

Bergler, R., Wechsung, S., Kienzle, E., Hoff, T. and Dobenecker, B. (2016) Nutrition consultation in small animal practice – a field for specialized veterinarians. *Tierarztl Prax Ausg K Kleintiere Heimtiere,* 44, 5–14.

Buchanan, R.L., Baker, R.C., Charlton, A.J., Riviere, J.E. and Standaert, R. (2011) Pet food safety: a shared concern. *British Journal of Nutrition,* 106, S78–S84.

Cake, M.A., Bell, M.A., Williams, J.C., Brown, F.J.L., Dozier, M. *et al.* (2016) Which professional (non-technical) competencies are most important to the success of graduate veterinarians? A Best Evidence Medical Education (BEME) systematic review: BEME Guide No. 38. *Medical Teacher,* 38(6), 550–563.

Chandler, M. (2018) Busting pet nutrition myths. *In Focus,* Available at: https://www.veterinary-practice.com/article/busting-pet-nutrition-myths (accessed 8 September 2022).

Churchill, J. and Ward, E. (2016) Communicating with pet owners about obesity: Roles of the veterinary health care team. *Veterinary Clinics of North America: Small Animal Practice,* 46(5), 899–911.

Clemens, R. (2014) The 'Humanization' of pet food. *Food Technology,* 8(14), 20.

Cline, M.G., Burns, K.M., Coe, J.B., Downing, R., Durzi, T. *et al.* (2021) 2021 AAHA nutrition and weight management guidelines for dogs and cats. *Journal of the American Animal Hospital Association,* 57(4), 153–178.

Coe, J.B, Adams, C.L, Eva, K, Desmarais, S. and Bonnett, B.N. (2010) Development and validation of an instrument for measuring appointment-specific client satisfaction in companion animal practice. *Preventative Veterinary Medicine,* 93, 201–210.

Davies, M. (2012) Geriatric screening in first opinion practice – results from 45 dogs. *Journal of Small Animal Practice,* 53(9), 507–513.

Dysart, L.M., Coe, J.B. and Adams, C.L. (2011) Analysis of solicitation of client concerns in companion animal practice. *Journal of the American Veterinary Medical Association,* 228, 1609–1615.

Finley, R., Reid-Smith, R., Ribble, C., Popa, M., Vandermeer, M. *et al.* (2008) The occurrence and antimicrobial susceptibility of salmonellae isolated from commercially available canine raw food diets in three Canadian cities. *Zoonoses and Public Health,* 55(8-10), 462–469.

Fitch, A.K. and Bays, H.E. (2022) Obesity definition, diagnosis, bias, standard operating procedures (SOPs), and telehealth: An Obesity Medicine Association (OMA) Clinical Practice Statement (CPS). *Obesity Pillars,* 1, 1–22.

Freeman, L.M., Chandler, M.L., Hamper, B.A. and Weeth, L.P. (2013). Current knowledge about the risks and benefits of raw meat-based diets for dogs and cats. *Journal of the American Veterinary Medical Association,* 243(11), 1549–1558.

Graafland, M., Schraagen, J.M.C., Boermeester, M.A., Bemelman, W.A. and Schijven, M.P. (2015) Training situational awareness to reduce surgical errors in the operating room. *British Journal of Surgery,* 102(1), 16–23.

Groat, E.F. Williams, N.J., Pinchbeck, G., Warner, B., Simpson, A. *et al.* (2022) UK dogs eating raw meat diets have higher risk of Salmonella and antimicrobial-resistant Escherichia colifaecal carriage. *Journal of Small Animal Practice,* 63(6), 435–441.

Hanford, R. and Linder, D.E. (2021) Impact of obesity on quality of life and owner's perception of weight loss programs in cats. *Veterinary Sciences,* 8(2), 1–6.

Heinze, C.R., Gomez, F.C. and Freeman, L.M. (2012) Assessment of commercial diets and recipes for home-prepared diets recommended for dogs with cancer. *Journal of the American Veterinary Medical Association,* 241(11), 1453–1460.

Hodgkiss, B.A., Lo, A.W.F., Loney, C.L., Wickers, A.S.J. and Yam, P.S. (2020) What's weighing on your mind? A novel approach to canine weight management. Presented at the 4th annual INSPIRE Research Forum, January 22, 2020, Glasgow, UK.

Ito, Y., Ishikawa, H., Suzuki, A. and Kato, M. (2022) The relationship between evaluation of shared decision-making by pet owners and veterinarians and satisfaction with veterinary consultations. *BMC Veterinary Research,* 18(296), 1–9.

Janke, N., Coe, J.B., Bernardo, T.M., Dewey, C.E. and Stone, E.A. (2021) Pet owners' and veterinarians' perceptions of information exchange and clinical decision-making in companion animal practice. *PLoS ONE,* 16(2): e0245632.

Janke, N., Shaw, J.R. and Coe, J.B. (2022) Veterinary technicians contribute to shared decision-making during companion animal veterinary appointments. *Journal of the American Veterinary Medical Association,* 260(15), 1993–2000.

Joffe, D.J. and Schlesinger, D.S., (2002) Preliminary assessment of the risk of Salmonella infection in dogs fed raw chicken diets. *Journal of the American Veterinary Medical Association,* 43, 441–442.

Kamleh, M., Khosa, D.K., Verbrugghe, A., Dewey, C.E. and Stone, E. (2020) A cross-sectional study of pet owners' attitudes and intentions towards nutritional guidance received from veterinarians. *Veterinary Record*, 187(12), e123.

Kanji, N., Coe, J.B., Adams, C.L. and Shaw, J.R. (2012) Effect of veterinarian-client-patient interactions on client adherence to dentistry and surgery recommendations in companion-animal practice. *Journal of the American Veterinary Medical Association*, 240(4), 427–436.

Kinnison, T., Guile, D. and May, S.A. (2015) Errors in veterinary practice: Preliminary lessons for building better veterinary teams. *The Veterinary Record*, 177(19), 492.

Kinnison, T. (2015) Insights from veterinary interprofessional interactions: Implications for interprofessional education (ipe) in the veterinary curricula. UCL Institute of Education. Available at: https://discovery.ucl.ac.uk/id/eprint/1495902/1/Thesis_Final.pdf (accessed 8 November 2022).

Kobayashi, H., Pian-Smith, M., Sato, M., Sawa, R., Takeshita, T. *et al.* (2006) A cross-cultural survey of residents' perceived barriers in questioning/challenging authority. *Quality & Safety in Health Care*, 15(4), 277–283.

Küper, A.M. and Merle, R. (2019) Being nice is not enough: Exploring relationship-centered veterinary care with structural equation modeling. A quantitative study on German pet owners' perception. *Frontiers in Veterinary Science*, 6(56), 1–16.

Larsen, J.A., Parks, E.M., Heinze, C.R. and Fascetti, A.J. (2012) Evaluation of recipes for home-prepared diets for dogs and cats with chronic kidney disease. *Journal of the American Veterinary Medical Association*, 240(5), 532–538.

Latham, C.E. and Morris, A. (2007) Effects of formal training in communication skills on the ability of veterinary students to communicate with clients. *Veterinary Record*, 160, 181–186.

Lingard, L., Espin, S., Whyte, S, Regehr, G., Baker, G. *et al.* (2004) Communication failures in the operating room: an observational classification of recurrent types and effects. *Quality and Safety in Health Care*, 13(5), 330–334.

Lue, T.W., Pantenburg, D.P. and Crawford, P.M. (2008) Impact of the owner-pet and client-veterinarian bond on the care that pets receive. *Journal of the American Veterinary Medical Association,* 232, 531–540.

Macdonald, J., Gray, C. and Robbé, I. (2021) The development of a Veterinary Nurse–Client Communication Matrix [version 1]. *MedEdPublish,* 10, 144.

Mellanby, R.J. and Herrtage, M.E. (2004). Survey of mistakes made by recent veterinary graduates. *Veterinary Record*, 155(24), 761–765.

Mossop, L., Gray, C., Blaxter, A., Gardiner, A., MacEachern, K. *et al.* (2015) Communication skills training: what the vet schools are doing. *Veterinary Record*, 176, 114–117.

Mulrooney, H. (2019) Obesity – learning from the crisis in people. *Veterinary Record,* 185(11), 349.

Nemser, S.M., Doran, T., Grabenstein, M., McConnell, T., McGrath, T. *et al.* (2014) Investigation of Listeria, Salmonella, and Toxigenic Escherichia coli in various pet foods. *Foodborne Pathogens and Disease*, 11(9), 706–709.

Newton, C., Shryane, N. and Pampaka, M. (2019) Cognitive dissonance, health and ethics: Towards a longitudinal study of evolving vegetarian motivations.

In: Vinnari, E. and Vinnari, M. (eds) *Sustainable Governance and Management of Food Systems: Ethical Perspectives*. Wageningen Academic Publishers, Wageningen, The Netherlands, pp. 347–352.

Nickels, B.M. and Feeley, T.H. (2018) Breaking bad news in veterinary medicine. *Health Communication*, 33(9), 1105–1113.

Nilsson, O. (2015) Hygiene quality and presence of ESBL-producing *Escherichia coli* in raw food diets for dogs. *Infection Ecology & Epidemiology*, 5, 28758.

Niza, N.M.R.E., Vilela, C.L. and Ferreira, L.M.A. (2003) Feline pansteatitis revisited: Hazards of unbalanced home made diets. *Journal of Feline Medicine and Surgery*, 5, 271–277.

Okuyama, A., Wagner, C. and Bijnen, B. (2014) Speaking up for patient safety by hospital-based health care professionals: A literature review. *BMC Health Services Research*, 14(1), 1–8.

Oxtoby, C., Ferguson, E., White, K. and Mossop, L. (2015) We need to talk about error: causes and types of error in veterinary practice. *Veterinary Record*, 177(17), 438.

Patterson, K., Grenny, J., McMillan, R. and Switzler, A. (2001) *Crucial conversations: Tools for talking when stakes are high*. McGraw-Hill, New York.

Pearl, R.L., Wadden, T.A., Bach, C., Leonard, S.M. and Michel, K.E. (2020) Who's a good boy? Effects of dog and owner body weight on veterinarian perceptions and treatment recommendations. *International Journey of Obesity*, 44, 2455–2464.

Pun, J.K.H. (2020) An integrated review of the role of communication in veterinary clinical practice. *BMC Veterinary Research*, 16(394), 1–14.

Reason, J. (2000) Human error: Models and management. *British Medical Journal*, 320(7237), 768–770.

Rujoiu, O. and Rujoju, V. (2016) Animal companion loss and the veterinarian-client relationship – exploratory study. *Journal of Psychology (Revista de Psihologie)*, 62(3), 211–226.

Russell, E., Mossop, L., Forbes, E. and Oxtoby, C. (2022). Uncovering the 'messy details' of veterinary communication: An analysis of communication problems in cases of alleged professional negligence. *Veterinary Record*, 190(3).

Schleicher, M., Cash, S.B. and Freeman, L.M. (2019) Determinants of pet food purchasing decisions. *Canadian Veterinary Journal*, 60(6), 644–650.

Schotte, U., Borchers, D., Wulff, C. and Geue L. (2007) Salmonella Montevideo outbreak in military kennel dogs caused by contaminated commercial feed, which was only recognized through monitoring. *Veterinary Microbiology*, 119(2-4), 316–323.

Schwappach, D., Sendlhofer, G., Häsler, L., Gombotz, V., Leitgeb, K. *et al.* (2018). Speaking up behaviors and safety climate in an Austrian university hospital. *International Journal for Quality in Health Care*, 30(9), 701–707.

Shaw, J.R., Adams, C.L., Bonnett, B.N., Larson, S. and Roter, D.L. (2012) Veterinarian satisfaction with companion animal visits. *Journal of the American Veterinary Medical Association*, 240, 832–841.

Siewert, B., Swedeen, S., Brook, O.R., Eisenberg, R L. and Hochman, M. (2018) Barriers to safety event reporting in an academic radiology department: Authority gradients and other human factors. *Radiology*, 288(3), 693–698.

Sontas, B.H., Schwendenwein, I. and Schafer-Soni, S. (2014) Primary anestrus due to dietary hyperthyroidism in a miniature pinscher bitch. *Canadian Veterinary Journal*, 55(8), 781–785.

Stiver, S.L., Frazier, K.S. and Mauel, M.J. (2003) Septicemic salmonellosis in two cats fed a raw-meat diet. *Journal of American Animal Hospital Association,* 39, 538–542.

Stockman, J., Fascetti, A.J., Kass, P.H. and Larsen, J.A. (2013) Evaluation of recipes of home-prepared maintenance diets for dogs. *Journal of the American Veterinary Medical Association,* 242(11), 1500–1505.

Strohmeyer, R.A., Morley, P.S., Hyatt, D.R., Dargatz, D.A., Scorza, V. *et al.* (2006) Evaluation of bacterial and protozoal contamination of commercially available raw meat diets for dogs. *Journal of the American Veterinary Medical Association,* 228, 537–542.

Sutherland, K.A., Coe, J.B. and O'Sullivan, T.L. (2022) Exploring veterinary professionals' perceptions of pet weight-related communication in companion animal veterinary practice. *Veterinary Record,* e1973.

Taylor-Adams, S. and Vincent, C. (n.d.) Systems analysis of clinical incidents: The London Protocol. Available at: https://www.imperial.ac.uk/media/imperial-college/medicine/surgery-cancer/pstrc/londonprotocol_e.pdf (accessed 8 November 2022).

van Bree, F.P.J., Bokken, G.C.A.M., Mineur, R., Franssen, F., Opsteegh, M. *et al.* (2018) Zoonotic bacteria and parasites found in raw meat-based diets for cats and dogs. *The Veterinary Record,* 182(2), 50.

VDS (Veterinary Defence Society) (2021) About VetSafe. Available at: https://www.thevds.co.uk/aboutvetsafe (accessed 26 October 2022).

Verbrugghe, A., Paepa, D., Verhaert, L., Saunders, J., Fritz, J. *et al.* (2011) Metabolic bone disease and hyperparathyroidism in an adult dog fed an unbalanced home-made diet. *Vlaams Diergeneeskundig Tijdschrift,* 80, 61–68.

Wachter, R. M. and Pronovost, P. J. (2009) Balancing 'No blame' with accountability in patient safety. *The New England Journal of Medicine,* 361(14), 1401–1406.

Wainwright, J., Millar, K.M. and White, G.A. (2022) Owners' views of canine nutrition, weight status and wellbeing and their implications for the veterinary consultation. *Journal of Small Animal Practice,* 63, 381–388.

Ward, E. (2022a) How to expand the pet food conversation. *Today's Veterinary Business,* 6(3), 12–15.

Ward, E. (2022b) How to not talk like a salesperson. *Today's Veterinary Business,* 6(4), 10–13.

Ward, E. (2022c) Consistency creates credibility. *Today's Veterinary Business,* 6(2), 14–17.

Weese, J.S., Rousseau, J. and Arroyo, L. (2005) Bacterial evaluation of commercial canine and feline raw diets. *Canadian Veterinary Journal,* 46, 513–516.

Wilson, S.A., Villaverde, C., Fascetti, A.J. and Larsen, J.A. (2019) Evaluation of the nutritional adequacy of recipes for home-prepared maintenance diets for cats. *Journal of the American Veterinary Medical Association,* 254(10), 1172–1179.

Yin, S. (2007) Clinical Report: Raw food diets. *Veterinary Forum,* 24(11).

Developing an interprofessional nutrition programme: Roles and responsibilities

8

Rachel Lumbis

Abstract

Nutritional assessment is fundamental to optimal patient care and requires collaboration of the veterinary healthcare team (VHCT) to determine the most appropriate method and route of delivery, the patient's nutrient and energy requirements, and feeding goals, and to ensure appropriate monitoring and follow-up care. Yet, as highlighted in previous chapters, there are barriers to VHCT engagement with clients about pet nutrition and disparity between pet caretakers' desire for, and the provision of, a veterinary nutritional recommendation. This chapter will discuss how clear definition of responsibilities, with appropriate delegation and utilisation of all members of the VHCT can help to ensure that all aspects of nutritional care are carried out, from initial assessment and dietary recommendations through to the delivery of prompt and targeted nutrition, accurate monitoring and provision of pet caretaker advice and support. It also emphasises the importance of direct client engagement and interaction using digital communication and virtual consultations to help facilitate easy accessibility of the VHCT to clients and minimise the compliance gap between nutritional recommendation and execution.

Ensuring a team approach to integrated nutritional care

The veterinary healthcare team (VHCT) has a central role as the expert source of information for appropriate pet nutrition. Each member of the team with whom the client interacts has fundamental involvement in providing nutrition advice, care, support and recommendations. However, in busy general practices, performing thorough nutritional consultations can be challenging (Lynch, 2012). As already outlined in Chapters 3, 4 and 6, there is a current disconnect between pet caretakers' desire for, and the provision of, a veterinary nutritional recommendation and, amid marketing, the veterinarian's voice can be further absent (Lynch, 2012; Alvarez *et al.*, 2022). While veterinarians are considered leading authorities on pet nutrition and healthcare

© Rachel Lumbis and Tierney Kinnison 2023. *An Interprofessional Approach to Veterinary Nutrition* (R. Lumbis and T. Kinnison)
DOI: 10.1079/9781800621107.0008

(Connolly *et al.*, 2014; Schleicher *et al.*, 2019; Alvarez *et al.*, 2022), a small, but significant, anti-vet sentiment is brewing (McCormack, 2019). To remain relevant and trusted by pet owners, it is essential to have a knowledgeable and empowered VHCT, the members of which can maximise their influence as pet health experts and provide sensible, balanced, pertinent and evidence-based nutritional advice to clients. 'No veterinary team will succeed when communication and teamwork are lacking' (Walsh, 2022, p. 58).

The ability to work with professionals to deliver collaborative patient-centred care is a critical element of professional practice. The competencies needed to work effectively in an interprofessional healthcare environment include:

- a willingness to collaborate
- effective communication
- mutual trust and respect
- conflict resolution
- contribution towards shared care plans and goal-setting
- understanding and appreciation of professional role and responsibility.

Challenges to interprofessional practice include stereotypical views, interprofessional prejudice and lack of recognition and career fulfilment. Furthermore, contrasting professional motivations for work can make understanding each other's actions challenging (Kinnison *et al.*, 2016). These challenges all reflect, to varying degrees, failures in emotional intelligence on both sides of the interprofessional team. Effective interprofessional communication and collaboration leads to a good team environment founded on respect, trust and mutual support and should seek to overcome such challenges (Kinnison *et al.*, 2016).

Historically, veterinarians have been positioned at the top of a hierarchical workplace structure and have taken responsibility for all actions in the veterinary practice (Kinnison *et al.*, 2014). While great geographic variation exists, there is increasing professional diversity and patient care no longer tends to rest solely with one veterinarian. In many countries, veterinary teams frequently consist of multiple veterinarians, veterinary nurses or technicians (hereafter referred to as VNs), other paraprofessionals, receptionists and administrators, all of whom contribute to the completion of patient- and client-oriented tasks (Kinnison and May, 2016). Relieving veterinarians of the pressures of jobs that can be completed by suitably qualified and competent colleagues enables completion of the work that only they are qualified to carry out. This has a direct and positive impact on the care received by pets and their owners, veterinary practice productivity and revenue, and demonstrates the expertise of the VHCT (Boatright, 2019; Abood and Verton-Shaw 2021).

Nutrition is an aspect of care that can be directed by the veterinarian and implemented by VNs, with the help of support staff, all of whom can act as nutritional counsellors and advocates. A nutritional assessment (NA), as described in the World Small Animal Veterinary Association (WSAVA) Nutritional Assessment Guidelines (Freeman *et al.*, 2011) and outlined in

Chapter 4, is the fifth vital assessment in the standard patient examination and a cornerstone of patient healthcare. Many aspects of an NA constitute part of a routine patient examination and should therefore be performed at every patient visit and require little additional time or cost, yet are not always recognised as such. Instead, conducting an NA is often viewed with trepidation amidst practical concerns such as higher caseloads (Du Marchie Sarvaas, 2022) and insufficient available time (Lynch, 2012). Other commonly cited barriers to completion include a perceived lack of practitioner knowledge and confidence, and patient need, particularly in healthy animals (Alvarez *et al.*, 2022). A consistent and detailed interprofessional approach with the involvement and effort of all members of the VHCT, and the pet caretaker, can facilitate successful integration of nutrition as the fifth vital assessment (Cline *et al.*, 2021). It is therefore essential to capitalise on the many opportunities available throughout the NA process to leverage and utilise the entire team.

The coronavirus pandemic has seen a surge in pet acquisition but decreased client visits to veterinary practices, forcing veterinary clinics and the VHCT to change the way in which they function, particularly with the introduction of telemedicine, telecommunication and virtual consultations. Utilising all members of the VHCT to offer a blend of services to clients, including the digital augmentation of consultations, and the ability to request appointments and order products online, can increase client care, interaction and loyalty, helping to provide convenience alongside expert care. This is of particular importance in nutritional care and, especially, in the follow-up of nutritional recommendations when ongoing, readily and easily accessible help, advice and support is required and sought-after, but pet caretakers may be unable or unwilling to make regular in-person visits to the practice (*Today's Veterinary Practice*, 2020).

Embracing professional roles to optimise nutritional assessment, recommendations and intake

Multifaceted clinical knowledge is required to enhance the quality of nutritional management, to optimise nutritional support according to the health and nutritional status of each individual animal and to avoid potential complications. With the rise in global pet obesity, increasing availability of pet food and inaccurate information sources, experienced guidance is more important than ever and can help to optimise veterinary care and clarify confusing pet food choices, while adding value to veterinary services (Lynch 2012; Cline *et al.*, 2021).

Advancing the central role of the VHCT as the expert source of information for optimal pet nutrition requires the commitment, engagement and involvement of all members of the team to develop a strong nutrition programme and client–practice bond (Table 8.1). 'Veterinary healthcare teams that understand and embrace clinical nutrition and demonstrate in-clinic behaviours consistent with that conviction will benefit not only patients and clients but also

Table 8.1. An illustration of the roles and responsibilities that all VHCT members play in the planning, implementation and evaluation of a veterinary practice nutrition programme. Please note these points are not exhaustive. Practices are encouraged to review and edit these accordingly for their own use. Author's own table.

PLANNING PHASE	
 Practice manager	• Ensure that the timing for implementation of a nutrition programme is optimal so that team members are able to focus on the new service and associated protocols, develop self-confidence, knowledge and skills (Britton, 2019). • Define the practice's nutrition protocol and feeding philosophy, and make nutrition a fifth vital assessment – a belief and culture in the practice (Lynch, 2012). This is essential for clinical consistency and for creating credibility and trust (Boatright, 2019; Ward, 2022). • Arrange a nutritional standards consensus meeting with every veterinarian, the practice manager and at least one member of the VN, patient care and reception/client care teams in attendance (Tassava, 2016).
 Practice manager, all veterinarians and at least one member of the VN, patient care and reception/ client care teams	• Gain a consensus and produce specifically delineated, written guidelines and a hospital policy regarding the practice's nutrition protocol and feeding philosophy that transcends brands (Tassava, 2016; Ward, 2022). Shepherd this into acceptance by the entire VHCT through clear and defined leadership and promotion of a team consensus (Ward, 2022). Adding compliance responsibilities to the job description of all team members promotes accountability and helps to improve compliance (AAHA, 2009b). • Determine the resources and materials that will help team members to educate and support clients (Tassava, 2016). • Make decisions based on the group's consistent recommendations. • Determine the cost of attending the practice's nutrition clinic/service. Consider capping the price for the first few months during the staff learning phase until it is established. • Schedule a team meeting to discuss the written practice nutrition protocol and promote the integration of nutrition into patient visits and care. • Provide a copy of the proposed nutrition protocol and feeding philosophy to team members for consideration prior to the meeting (Ward, 2022).

Continued

Table 8.1. Continued.

PLANNING PHASE

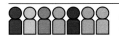

All members of the VHCT

At the team meeting
- Discuss the WSAVA Nutritional Assessment Guidelines and acknowledge the importance of including nutrition as the fifth vital assessment in the standard patient examination.
- Review and discuss the practice's written nutrition protocol and feeding philosophy. Gain a consensus and agree on certain foundational principles. 'Protocols that reflect input from every member of the practice team will be supported by every member of the team' (AAHA, 2009b, p. 9).
- Ensure that all members acknowledge the:
  - importance of communicating preventive nutrition to every client at every pet visit
  - commitment needed by everyone to provide consistent messages and a 'one voice' approach to veterinary nutrition to help create credibility and promote compliance (Ward, 2022)
  - need for civility and a desire for collaboration between all members of the VHCT and with pet caretakers (Ward, 2022.)
- Identify how to raise pet caretakers' awareness of the importance of nutrition.
- Identify how each team member will reinforce, implement and follow-up on dietary recommendations. Define the roles and responsibilities of each team member, including an outline of the tasks and procedures to be performed (Pet Nutrition Alliance, 2018). Individual level of competence, expertise, skills and knowledge should be considered.
- Review the questions that will be asked to obtain/verify the patient's diet history and to instigate a nutritional assessment (Lynch, 2012) – for example, 'What are you currently feeding and why?' (Ograin, 2016).
- Identify, train and utilise a motivated veterinary professional who is passionate about nutrition and enjoys communicating with clients to act as nutrition 'champion'. Responsibilities will include promoting the inclusion of nutrition as a standard component of patient care and reinforcing good nutritional practice throughout the veterinary clinic (Creevy *et al.*, 2019). Therefore, an enthusiasm for helping and educating is essential.

During/following the team meeting
- Encourage team members to identify any nutrition-related questions, reservations or clients' concerns they may have, so these can be addressed (Lynch, 2012).

Continued

Table 8.1. Continued.

PLANNING PHASE

Practice manager
Nutrition champion
Veterinarians

- Identify nutrition and communication-related training needs of the VHCT, including the nutrition 'champion'. All team members should undergo thorough training on the key points of the practice's philosophy on nutrition. This should include fundamental nutrition concepts and the diet products (therapeutic and non-therapeutic) stocked in the practice (Lynch, 2012). The VHCT should also be taught the science behind nutritional recommendations, assessment of body and muscle condition scoring, and calculation of basic daily caloric recommendations (Ward, 2022). Educating staff is key to any successful clinic programme (Buzhardt, 2003).

Ensure that the practice's written guidelines and hospital policy regarding the nutritional programme is communicated (ideally verbally and in written format) to all VHCT members, especially those who missed the team meeting.

IMPLEMENTATION PHASE

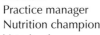

Practice manager
Nutrition champion
Office staff

- Coordinate and schedule regular in-clinic training that focuses on nutrition fundamentals for all team members and ensure the completion of appropriate continuing professional development (CPD) and continuing education (CE) for veterinarians and VNs. Role-play exercises and question-and-answer sessions can be particularly valuable for communication skills training and to help determine if team members' client communications are consistent with the expected standards (Donnelly, 2022) and aligned to the practice's nutrition protocol and feeding philosophy.
- The provision of in-clinic training focusing specifically on the consistent assessment and recording of body condition score (BCS) and muscle condition score (MCS) is crucial. Abood and Verton-Shaw (2021) recommend a frequency of two to three times per year.
- Encourage the VHCT to feed the practice's recommended pet foods.

Practice manager
Nutrition champion
Reception/client
 care team
Office staff

- Liaise with the VHCT to ensure the diets, treats and supplements ordered/stocked in the practice are sufficient to complement the nutritional recommendations being made. This can help to generate profit and enhance the client–practice bond (Lynch, 2012).

Continued

Table 8.1. Continued.

IMPLEMENTATION PHASE

Nutrition champion

- Invite patients that have recently undergone a neutering procedure for a 'complimentary' nutrition consultation with the nutrition champion or member of the VN team within a month of the surgery. The cost can be factored into the surgical procedure and would enable a discussion with the pet's caretaker about any necessary dietary modifications and the prevention of weight gain (Abood and Verton-Shaw, 2021).
- Communicate with the VHCT to ensure that all members feel empowered and sufficiently confident and knowledgeable to advocate optimal pet nutrition and to provide nutrition and diet-related support and education to pet caretakers.
- Ensure that all members of the VHCT acknowledge the importance of communicating preventive nutrition to every client at every pet visit.
- Review the nutrition-related educational materials available to pet caretakers on the practice's website and social media sites. Consider if there is scope for further development, such as the provision of nutrition-related blogs, videos and sound bites (Abood and Verton-Shaw, 2021).
- Display copies of commonly used, and ideally non-branded, nutritional tools, such as BCS, MCS, faecal score charts, nutritional assessment checklists and calorie requirements for healthy adult dogs and cats, to help facilitate nutrition discussions (Abood and Verton-Shaw, 2021; WSAVA, 2021).

Nutrition champion
Reception/client
  care team
Office staff

- Advertise the practice's nutrition programme and nutrition support service/clinic to pet caretakers and clients using a variety of methods, including visual displays, email/text messaging, leaflet drops and social media (John, 2022).
- Identify suitable patients to showcase and promote the nutrition support service/clinic. Create posters of patients to display in waiting areas and consultation rooms (Abood and Verton-Shaw, 2021).

Veterinarians
VN team
Nutrition champion

- Design or identify relevant documentation that will be used for nutritional care to hospitalised and non-hospitalised patients. Chapter 3 provides suggestions of credible and freely available resources.
- Identify common client nutrition questions or issues encountered during regular examinations. Develop written position statements to address these and/or identify relevant documentation that can be used for client educational purposes (Lynch, 2012).

Continued

Table 8.1. Continued.

IMPLEMENTATION PHASE

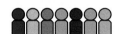

All members of the
VHCT

- Educate and encourage clients to participate in the nutritional assessment of their pet. Provide support with any necessary dietary modifications (Freeman *et al.*, 2011).
- Provide a list of alternative recommendations to the pet food stocked in the practice, including grocery options. This helps to ensure the practice's nutrition support service/clinic is helpful and inclusive, while still emphasising and promoting the importance of optimal pet health (Lynch, 2012).
- Consider ways of reaching out and promoting nutritional assessments and nutrition conversations to clients who cannot, or do not, make regular visits to the practice. For example, by hosting a nutrition-focused online client education event.
- Ensure consistent use of screening tools and criteria to make nutritional assessments of all patients and pets at every visit. Record results on patient records and ensure accountability for the identification of malnutrition.
- All staff members should acknowledge the importance of nutrition in veterinary care. This can be enhanced by involving the dedicated nutrition champion in (interdisciplinary) patient rounds and in-house staff training sessions.
- Ensure that all team members are positive and enthusiastic about the nutrition programme and associated services. Team buy-in and personal belief is needed for natural promotion to pet caretakers (Britton, 2019).
- Encourage effective teamwork with appropriate colleague referral to the practice's nutrition clinic/ services and effective utilisation of the nutrition champion (Corbee, 2019). If appropriate, ensure referral to a Board-Certified Veterinary Nutritionist.
- Ensure that any appointments with the nutrition support service/clinic are documented and appear on the schedule, like any other appointment with a veterinarian or VN.
- Try and ensure continuity of nutritional care, where possible. Pairing each patient with the nutrition champion or another individual veterinary professional can help to build client trust, reduce pet fear and enhance both the client–practice bond and the team member's role (Cline *et al.*, 2021).

Continued

Table 8.1. Continued.

EVALUATION PHASE

Practice manager
Nutrition champion
Veterinarians

- According to the American Animal Hospital Association (AAHA) (2009b, p. 27), sustainability depends on three critical components:
  1. ongoing and frequent staff training
  2. monitoring and reporting results
  3. continuing commitment on the part of the practice leadership.
- Communicate with the VHCT to ensure that all members *continue* to:
  o feel empowered to advocate for optimal pet nutrition
  o provide consistent nutrition and diet-related support and education to pet caretakers
  o consistently promote the veterinary practice's nutrition policies and feeding philosophy
  o demonstrate passion for nutritional assessment and enthusiasm when making dietary recommendations (Ward, 2022).
- Conduct client communications training for specific team members. Donnelly (2022) recommends a duration and frequency of 15–30 minutes at least twice per week and emphasises the importance of overcoming the mindset of 'I don't have time to train' to ensure that pets receive the care they deserve and that clients expect.
- Provide a suggestion box with well designed suggestion slips, prompting the provision of constructive feedback from staff and clients on the practice's nutrition service and associated protocols.
- Review the number of patients engaging with the practice's nutrition support service/clinic and the level of client satisfaction.
- Review the number of patients being given a nutritional recommendation and ensure that these are being followed up.
- Ensure that a consistent message in relation to the practice's philosophy on nutrition is being maintained in all areas of the practice.
- Evaluate the cost of attending the practice's nutrition clinic/service. Ensure it is still appropriate and financially viable.
- Compliment staff on their team effort as well as recognising the excellence and accomplishments of individual team members (Buzhardt, 2003).

Continued

Table 8.1. Continued.

EVALUATION PHASE

Nutrition champion
VN team
Veterinarians
Patient care
  assistants

- Ensure the nutrition champion's involvement in (interdisciplinary) patient rounds and in-house nutrition-related training for the entire VHCT.
- Identify whether nutritional recommendations are being documented in patients' medical records. Is there evidence of collaborative planning of nutritional care, with input from owners and colleagues?
- Review the daily monitoring of hospitalised patients to ensure that nutritional assessment items, such as BCS, MCS, body weight, feeding orders, fluid balance and diet/nutrient intake, are being accurately and consistently recorded.

Practice manager
Nutrition champion
Reception/client care
  team
Office staff

- Review the diets, treats and supplements being ordered/stocked in the practice and ensure these are sufficient to complement the nutritional recommendations being made.
- Ensure that the nutrition champion has ordering privileges for issues relating to nutritional support and care.

their practice and the profession' (Cline *et al.*, 2021, p. 170). Benefits of employing a team healthcare and patient-centred delivery model of veterinary care with utilisation of the entire VHCT include:

- increasing pet caretakers' access to, and time spent with, a veterinary professional
- provision of an integrated, cohesive message promoting the importance of nutrition and the value of optimal animal health and preventive pet care, including nutrition
- maximising the effectiveness of pet food recommendations, helping to reduce the compliance gap between recommendations and execution (Hancock and Schubert, 2007; Gerrard, 2015)
- enhancing the client–pet and client–practice relationship
- promotion of a long-term client relationship with the practice
- increased efficiency and alleviation of unbalanced workloads through more even distribution of work (Cline *et al.*, 2021; Carter and Grant, 2022)
- provision of greater job satisfaction and staff retention (Boatright, 2019)
- increased morale and motivation (Cline *et al.*, 2021)
- promotion of team contribution to success
- substantial rise in productivity (Lester, 2021) and increased revenue for the hospital (Cline *et al.*, 2021).

Ensuring a coherent approach to the maintenance of the health and well-being of animals committed to our care should be of paramount importance and involve the delegation of work according to relevant skills, competence and expertise. It is important to identify which team members are responsible for nutritional assessment, planning, intervention and reinforcing recommendations. By reviewing each stage of a patient's visit to the practice, it is possible to identify ways to leverage different members of the VHCT (Table 8.2).

A VN-led nutrition service

Not all practices have the luxury of VNs or VN-led clinics, but these can be invaluable in supporting clinical practice (John, 2022), particularly in providing preventative nutrition (Verton-Shaw, 2016) and discussing the often-neglected topic of nutrition for healthy animals (Lynch, 2012). As identified by Cline *et al.*, (2021, p. 170), 'The veterinary technician is poised to lead the initiative to provide nutritional care for all patients'. Nutrition is a critical component of caring for and treating small animals and one in which VNs and support staff play a key role. Alongside veterinarians, VNs are frequently identified as a source of nutrition advice and recommendations to pet owners (Bruckner and Handl, 2020; Lumbis and de Scally 2020; Blees *et al.*, 2021) and can have a positive impact on owners' understanding of nutritional recommendations (Freeman *et al.*, 2011; Johnson and Linder 2013). Their skills and knowledge are critical to assisting veterinarians with the nutritional assessment process, formulation of feeding plans and provision of necessary nutritional support (Chan and Freeman, 2006) as well as being proficient at nutritional consulting (Shock *et al.*, 2020). It is therefore important that the views of VNs are considered when implementing nutrition as a vital assessment in small animal practice. It should also be the joint responsibility of veterinarians and the VN team to ensure the early identification of animals in need of nutritional support. Once dietary modification or nutritional intervention is deemed necessary, collaboration is essential to determine the most appropriate method and route of delivery, alongside establishment of the patient's nutrient needs and feeding goals (Freeman *et al.*, 2011). 'The best practices formulate treatment plans with both veterinarians and VNs' (Yagi, 2017, p. 23).

The legal scope of a VN's practice varies according to geographic location and is usually defined by country or state, with the provision of a diagnosis and prognosis, prescription of medications and completion of surgical procedures generally limited to veterinarians (Yagi, 2017). Despite their rigorous training and critical role, many veterinary practices fail to recognise and appreciate the extensive skills and potential of VNs, contributing to underutilisation and underappreciation (Yagi, 2017; Boatright, 2019; Chadwick, 2022). In the UK, registered veterinary nurses (RVNs) are regulated professionals who are responsible for adhering to a code of professional conduct (RCVS, 2022) and are subject to a disciplinary system. If a task is appropriately delegated to an

Table 8.2. Identification of the role and responsibilities that different members of the VHCT can assume in relation to nutritional assessment, care and support at each stage of a pet's visit to the veterinary practice. Please note these points are not exhaustive. Practices are encouraged to review and edit these accordingly for their own use. Author's own table.

1. Pre-appointment and obtaining a dietary history

Veterinary practice
Practice manager

- Is the practice using all available methods of communication to invite clients to bring their pet in for a nutritional assessment and discussion about diet? Is it making the most of opportunities to share trusted and evidence-based nutrition information with clients using the practice's website, app and social media sites, as well as other communication tools such as email and text? It is important to normalise conversations about nutrition for those clients coming to the practice as well as those who make rare visits or infrequent contact.
- In addition to publishing photos of visiting pets and patients, does the veterinary practice feature images of, and a brief biography for, all team members on its web and social media sites? This can prompt feelings of familiarity and help to enhance the human–animal bond (HAB) and relationship between practice, VHCT, clients and patients (*Today's Veterinary Practice*, 2020). It also helps to promote the interprofessional VHCT which is important for clients to see and understand and can be used to highlight expertise and special interests that team members may have, such as nutrition (Kinnison, 2017).
- For those patients with an upcoming appointment, does the practice make use of a diet history form?
- If appointment reminders are being sent out, consider including a message to highlight the importance of nutrition. Request that clients bring with them, or submit online in advance, digital pictures of food products, rewards and supplements being given to their pet (Abood and Verton-Shaw, 2021).
- The internet and social media are common sources of information for many pet caretakers. Consider ways of engaging clients in conversations about what they have learned prior to the appointment and direct them to reliable resources (Janke *et al.*, 2021).

Reception/client
care team
Office staff

- Can the administration or reception team facilitate a pet caretaker's completion of a diet history form at home by phoning the client or sending an email or text link? A clear and brief accompanying explanation of why this information is being obtained and requested prior to the pet's appointment is crucial.

Continued

Table 8.2. Continued.

---

2. Welcome in clinic and revisiting and emphasising previous recommendations

Reception/client
care team

Does the reception team do the following?

• Facilitate pet caretakers' completion of a pre-visit questionnaire, including a diet history form, sent by email, text message or direct web link before their pet's appointment? Ideally, this will have been completed at home and submitted prior to arrival.

• Utilise weighing scales in the waiting area to obtain an accurate body weight of canine patients and record it appropriately.

• Ask questions about diet history at every patient visit so that caretakers anticipate nutrition-related questions and come prepared with sufficient information to answer these (Abood and Verton-Shaw, 2021).

• Review the pet's medical records, identify any previous dietary recommendations made by the veterinarian or VN and highlight/discuss these with the caretaker to get an update on compliance? 'A simple compliance checklist, in the hands of proactive team members, can yield great results for the practice – and the pets it serves' (AAHA, 2009b, p. 16).

• Ask clients for their permission to send basic updates about their pet and appointment/healthcare reminders via text messaging and email.

• Prompt caretakers to download the practice's app or follow the practice on social media for easily accessible, reliable and evidence-based pet nutrition and healthcare information.

Veterinary practice
Practice manager

• Is the practice team embracing all available opportunities to provide visual awareness of the importance of nutrition in waiting areas, including the use of flat screens and poster displays (John, 2022)?

• Does the practice's computer software facilitate easy recording of nutritional assessment data with appropriate triggers in place for initiating the next steps if suboptimal results are obtained?

3. Nutritional assessment and obtaining a dietary history

VN team

• Is there the space and time available for a VN to obtain a body weight and to assess the pet's body and muscle condition score?

• Are they also able to obtain a complete dietary history and identify any nutrition-related concerns/queries from the caretaker?

• Is this information being accurately recorded in the patient's records?

Continued

Table 8.2. Continued.

---

4. Nutritional recommendation by the veterinarian

Veterinarians

- Are the veterinarians able to utilise the dietary history and patient information obtained prior to the appointment, along with further questioning, diagnostics and results of a patient examination, to make a nutritional recommendation?
- Is the nutritional recommendation and plan being documented in the pet's medical records? This is essential, even if only to confirm the timing of the next visit/follow-up (AAHA, 2009b). Use of the SOAP (subjective, objective, assessment and plan) format can help to ensure the documentation of critical information in a swift, clear and organised layout (Table 8.3).
- Is the pet at the centre of the nutritional recommendation? Are owners being given a clear explanation regarding how and why the recommendation will benefit their pet's health and wellbeing? This can help to improve compliance (AAHA, 2010).
- Is there sufficient available time for clients to ask questions? Have they been given a chance to contribute to the nutritional plan? Are they making an informed choice for their pet?

5. Hospital admission (if applicable)

Nutrition champion
Veterinarians
VNs
Patient care
 assistants
Reception/client
 care team

- Which team members are responsible for admitting patients to the hospital?
- Is there an opportunity for VNs, patient care assistants or the reception/client care team to question caretakers about their pet's usual dietary regime and feeding habits/predilections as part of a wider survey into their pet's normal daily routine and preferences?
- If yes, is this information being recorded on the patient's records?

6. Hospitalisation (if applicable)

Nutrition champion
Veterinarians
VNs
Patient care
 assistants
Reception/client
 care team

- Which team members have responsibility for administering nutritional support to patients and monitoring food intake? Is the practice's nutrition policy being followed? Are readily available tools being utilised, such as the WSAVA's guides and charts?
- How are feeding orders communicated to team members? Is this clear, transparent and effective?
- Are the energy requirements of hospitalised patients being met? Where and how is this information being recorded?

Continued

Table 8.2. Continued.

- Are the skills of patient care assistants being fully utilised to support food provision and ensure the accurate monitoring of dietary intake? Are they also supporting the VN team in monitoring patients and identifying changes to aspects such as elimination, food intake, demeanour and behaviour? Where and how is this information being recorded?
- Is nutrition being considered and discussed during patient handovers?
- Are caretakers being kept informed of their pet's care and progress? Is it the same member of the vet and/or VN team who is making contact? Is there evidence of consistency in the information being provided?

7. Hospital discharge (if applicable) or check out at reception

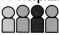

Nutrition champion
VN team
Patient care
  assistants
Reception/client
  care team

- Is the veterinarian's recommendation being supported and further explained to the client, with clear emphasis on how and why it will impact on the pet's health and wellbeing? Providing appropriate levels of information, together with a summary of what was said during the consultation, can facilitate understanding (Little, 2013). However, for compliance to succeed, pet caretakers need to accept and agree with the recommendation rather than simply being told what it is (AAHA, 2009b).
- Are pet caretakers given specific verbal and written instructions, including a summary of the nutrition recommendation and plan? Reinforcing verbal communication with other educational materials can help to ensure compliance and consistency in the message delivered by the VHCT.
- Are all members of the VHCT confident in calculating the daily cost to feed the recommended diet? Therapeutic diets can be more expensive than many over-the-counter products but, in the case of ultra-premium grocery brands, not always. It is also important to highlight the positive effect that the recommended diet can have on quality and length of life, disease progression or prevention and potential cost of veterinary care.
- Are follow-up appointments being scheduled to reassess the pet's body weight and condition, and to follow up on adherence to nutritional recommendations? Compliance can only be achieved when the nutritional recommendation is well accepted by the client and followed through (AAHA, 2009a; Corbee, 2019).

Continued

Table 8.2. Continued.

Veterinary practice
Practice manager

- Have appropriate and efficient reminder systems been implemented, together with the establishment of clear standard operating procedures and rigorous processes that all team members buy into? This is fundamental to creating, reinforcing, reminding/supporting and following up on nutritional recommendations (Little, 2013).
- Is it possible to customise the practice's software, enabling automatic periodic reminders to be sent out to clients, reminding them to bring their pet for a nutritional assessment and discussion about diet (*Today's Veterinary Practice*, 2020)?

8. Follow-up phone/video call to provide support and encouragement, and check compliance/adherence to recommendations (two to three days later)

Veterinary practice
Practice manager

- After the initial nutritional recommendation, follow-up calls should be scheduled for two to three days, two weeks and two months to see how the pet is doing (Ograin, 2016). The relationship with a client doesn't end when they leave the practice, therefore continuing the conversation is crucial to nurture the bond between client, practice and VHCT (Walsh, 2022). It also reiterates to the pet caretaker the importance the practice places on nutritional recommendations, which is essential for increasing compliance (Corbee, 2019).
- Depending on the individual pet and dietary plan, the frequency of contact may need to be modified. For example, if weight loss is recommended, caretakers should be called at least monthly, and pets should be weighed at least every two to four weeks until they reach the desired weight (Ograin, 2016).
- Is it easy for pet caretakers to make an online request for an appointment with the nutrition champion or a veterinary professional or to easily contact the VHCT or nutrition champion via web chat/video chat/messenger? Pet caretakers need to know someone is there for them to help with questions or concerns (Ograin, 2016), otherwise they may abandon the dietary plan (Lynch, 2012).
- Where possible, is there continuity of contact and an emotional connection between clients and the practice? Are clients and their pets being paired with a specific team member? Repeating information and continued questioning can be frustrating and off-putting for clients who desire clear, timely and personal communication (*Vet Times*, 2022).

Continued

Table 8.2. Continued.

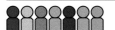

All members of the
VHCT

- Is the entire practice team on board with compliance protocols? Is there consistency among team members?
- Are team members well versed in encouraging repeat visits and follow-up appointments/calls? This is important to ensure concordance and compliance (Little, 2013), but also to be an advocate for the pet and caretaker (Ograin, 2016).

VNs
Patient care
  assistants
Reception/client
  care team
Nutrition champion

- Which team members have responsibility for following up on nutritional recommendations with clients? Are they doing this? If so, are multiple approaches to client communication being used, such as phone call, text message and email, or alternative methods?
- Are they proactive? Do they check-in with clients regularly and make repeated contact attempts if there is no answer or response? Making follow-up phone calls to unresponsive clients improves compliance (AAHA, 2009a).

Nutrition champion
VNs

- Was a feeding plan provided, either electronically or in hard copy, when the nutritional recommendation was originally made? If not, the nutrition champion or one of the VNs should provide this. It is of particular value if a dietary change is being recommended, including changes in the provision of treats and supplements, and should briefly outline the:
  ○ exact diet being recommended and why
  ○ diet features and relevance for the patient and client
  ○ precise amount to be fed and frequency (Verton-Shaw, 2016).
- Discuss with the client any issues that may limit adherence to dietary recommendations (e.g., clients' time/lifestyle and feeding schedule issues, complex instructions and financial limitations) and address these accordingly.

9. Follow-up call with client or attendance at nutrition support clinic to check body weight/condition, provide support and encouragement and check compliance levels (two to three weeks later)

Nutrition champion
VNs

- Is the nutrition champion or a member of the VN team calling clients after two to three weeks following the initial visit and nutrition recommendation? Are clients attending the nutrition support clinic for a follow-up appointment with their pet?
- Is the pet's body weight, BCS and MCS being assessed as part of a more thorough nutritional assessment? Are these details being recorded?
- Is the nutritional recommendation and feeding plan being reviewed and verified with the client? Are goals and dietary portioning being adjusted as required?

Continued

Table 8.2. Continued.

Nutrition champion
VNs
Veterinarians

Practice manager
Nutrition champion
VNs
Reception/client
   care team
Veterinary practice

- Are questions from the client being actively encouraged and answered? It is important for the team member to empathise and talk through any struggles that clients are facing with their pet or the recommended diet. Trust, logic and clarity of communication and information provision can further increase the chance of compliance (Gerrard, 2015).
- If the client expresses concern with the nutritional plan and demonstrates a lack of willingness to adhere, it may be appropriate to refer the conversation back to the original veterinarian or discuss with them any potential modifications that can be made.
- Are future nutritional assessment and follow-up appointments being scheduled? Is it easy for pet caretakers to book future appointments online, via the practice's webpage, social media, online app or an alternate platform?

10. Follow-up phone/video call to provide support and encouragement, and check if more food is needed (two to three months later)

Veterinary practice
Practice manager

Nutrition champion

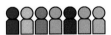

All members of the
   VHCT

Reception/client care
   team
Office staff

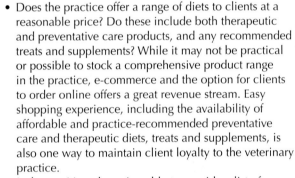

- Does the practice offer a range of diets to clients at a reasonable price? Do these include both therapeutic and preventative care products, and any recommended treats and supplements? While it may not be practical or possible to stock a comprehensive product range in the practice, e-commerce and the option for clients to order online offers a great revenue stream. Easy shopping experience, including the availability of affordable and practice-recommended preventative care and therapeutic diets, treats and supplements, is also one way to maintain client loyalty to the veterinary practice.
- Is the nutrition champion able to provide a list of alternative recommendations to the food stocked in the practice, including supermarket brands? This can help to address the needs and desires of all clients, making the practice's nutrition service helpful and inclusive.
- Are team members encouraged to feed the practice's recommended pet foods? Feeding *their* pets the food they recommend is the best endorsement to clients (Lynch, 2012).
- An inventory/office manager or member of the reception team is perfectly placed to make regular calls to caretakers to enquire how their pet is and to ascertain if more food is needed.

Table 8.3. An example of use of the SOAP (subjective, objective, assessment, and plan) format to document critical information from the nutritional assessment, plan and recommendation in a swift, clear and organised layout. Author's own table.

S	Bilateral TPLO (tibial plateau levelling osteotomy) surgery performed six weeks ago due to cruciate ligament disease.
	Restricted exercise, increased treat provision and same food intake during recovery period contributing to weight gain.
O	Body weight: 32.6 kg; BCS: 8/9; MCS: normal.
	Confined to room rest (daytime) or crate rest (overnight) and lead exercise only.
A	Body weight was 10% over optimum at time of surgery.
	Current body weight is 15% over optimum.
	Recovery progressing well and exercise can be gradually increased over the next four weeks.
P	Arrange in-person or video/phone appointment with nutrition champion within one to two days to discuss an appropriate reduction in calorie intake and gradual increase in exercise.

RVN, they become professionally responsible and accountable for its completion. This is different to many other countries where the veterinarian retains full responsibility for the delegatee's acts or omissions and overall outcome. Appropriate delegation of work according to relevant skills, competence and expertise, rather than hierarchical status, can help to promote more efficient and cost-effective patient care. It also contributes to greater job satisfaction, respect, appreciation and recognition. Robust professional communication and accurate record-keeping is needed to enhance and support delegation, thus promoting a united VHCT and high-quality patient, and client, care. This is key to the provision of nutritional support and all other aspects of veterinary care and treatment.

In general practice, a dedicated VN, who is well trained and passionate about nutrition, could set up a nutrition clinic/service and act as nutritional champion, not only for their own practice but potentially also for other committed local practices (Corbee, 2019). When utilised in this way, VNs can potentiate their value by improving patient outcomes and care (*Veterinary Practice*, 2020), enhancing client experience, expectations and satisfaction, increasing practice productivity (Lynch, 2012; Corbee, 2019) and enhancing the client–practice bond (John, 2022), thus promoting client loyalty and compliance (Gerrard, 2015). Several other intrinsic and economic benefits can be gained through appropriate delegation to a VN and the provision of a VN-led nutrition service/clinic, including:

- Provision of more time and cost-effective care, freeing up vets' time to complete the tasks only they are qualified to perform (Shock *et al.*, 2020; Lester, 2021). Improved efficiency and streamlining of workflow are of particular importance in the post-pandemic era as veterinarians juggle an increasingly complex and remote patient load, and pet caretakers start scheduling more appointments (Chadwick, 2022).

- Strengthening the bond between patient and VN, and client and VN, therefore helping caretakers to fulfil their responsibilities to their pet (Wiggins, 2016).
- Increased revenue generation and practice profitability (Lynch, 2012; Corbee, 2019; Shock *et al.*, 2020), with income and value directly attributed to an increased level of formally trained and educated support personnel (Fanning and Shepherd, 2010; Yagi, 2017; AVMA, 2022).
- Pet caretaker compliance has been known to increase when education and recommendations are delivered by non-veterinarians (Hancock and Schubert, 2007).
- VNs spend a significant amount of time interacting with pets and communicating with and supporting caretakers, potentially more than a veterinarian does. This helps to build relationships and trust, as well as increasing client compliance and satisfaction (Walsh, 2022)
- Maximising the effectiveness of pet food recommendations by:
  - helping pet caretakers to understand the underpinning reasons for the recommendation given, increasing the chances of acceptance and approval (Walsh, 2022) – owners are often willing to follow nutritional recommendations, particularly if they understand the benefit to their pets' health (AAHA, 2010)
  - increasing the time spent with a veterinary professional through use of reminder systems, text or direct messaging for client communication and video chat
  - providing timely encouragement (Hancock and Schubert, 2007; Gerrard, 2015)
  - encouraging clients to ask questions and clarifying any queries they may have – not all pet caretakers understand everything they are told, and many are reluctant or uncomfortable asking questions (Walsh, 2022).
- Pet caretakers are more likely to disclose information to a VN because they feel too embarrassed or uncomfortable speaking to a veterinarian (Yeates, 2014) or they do not want to bother them (Gerrard, 2015) or waste their time (Yeates, 2014). This can include the provision of a more detailed and accurate dietary history. Many clients also feel less conscious of time and are therefore more at ease to discuss any concerns and ask for advice from a VN (Wiggins, 2016).
- Greater development of the VN's role with enhanced job satisfaction, respect, appreciation and recognition, leading to happier colleagues (Boatright, 2021) and a greater chance of staff retention (Chadwick, 2022).
- Educating pet caretakers and addressing their misconceptions about the role, responsibilities, education and skills of a VN, thus promoting greater public recognition, respect and understanding of the VN's role (Writer-Davies, 2019; *Today's Veterinary Nurse*, 2022).

Many potential opportunities exist for VNs to raise awareness of the importance of optimal pet nutrition and to discuss diet with caretakers (Fig. 8.1)

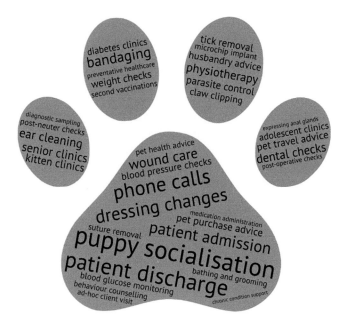

Fig. 8.1. An example of the opportunities available for VNs to raise awareness of the importance of optimal pet nutrition and to discuss diet with caretakers. Created using https://wordart.com/. Word size is randomised and bears no significance. Author's own figure.

but success of a VN-led nutrition clinic is reliant on effective interprofessional teamwork, support and communication. It also requires:

- A dedicated VN (or, ideally, a nutrition champion) who is enthusiastic about nutrition, well trained and has excellent communication skills.
- Sufficient time for nutrition consultations and nutrition training (Corbee, 2019).
- The availability of physical space – there should be a dedicated area for the nutrition service, so the VN is able to chat with a client without being disturbed, and has a display of tools (bags, treats, feeding toys, anatomy models, charts, weighing scales and books).
- Awareness by veterinarians (and all staff members) of the existence of the nutrition clinic, with a willingness to support this and make referrals when appropriate. Traditional hierarchical structures may be challenged and communication problems can occur, both of which need to be considered and overcome.
- A structure that enables the same level of service provision to be maintained, irrespective of the individual delivering the clinic. Consistency in process and information delivery promotes a positive client experience and builds confidence in the ability of the VHCT (Hollwarth and Vickery, 2022).

- Acknowledgement, acceptance and promotion by the veterinary practice and all staff members of the important role that VNs play and their associated financial value. 'A practice that utilises VNs at the highest level can empower them with autonomy' (Yagi, 2017, p. 23).
- A value attached to the VN's skills, knowledge and professional time, with the VN clinic being charged for accordingly (Writer-Davies, 2019; Hollwarth and Vickery, 2022). In contrast to consultations with a veterinarian, a VN's time, work and responsibilities are often charged through procedure or service. For example, care of feeding tubes, urinalysis, dental scale and polish, monitoring anaesthesia, placing catheters and microchips and administering medication and second vaccinations. It is therefore not always obvious (*Veterinary Practice*, 2020) and invoicing is rarely transparent to reflect a VN's contribution to patient care (Writer-Davies, 2019). Registered VNs and technicians are expertly trained and highly skilled and knowledgeable veterinary professionals who provide a necessary and valuable service for animals and their caretakers (Shock *et al.*, 2020; RCVS, 2022). The value of charging for VN clinics can generate revenue otherwise missed (*Veterinary Practice*, 2020) and bring more respect, benefits and value for money for the client (Hollwarth and Vickery, 2022).

Encouraging and enabling VNs to provide nutrition-focused clinics is one strategy that can take advantage of their proficiency, motivate pet caretakers to seek expert advice on diet and feeding management and, ultimately, influence positive patient outcomes, enhance client satisfaction and contribute to practice revenue. However, functionality must be predicated on positive relationships between colleagues, appropriate utilisation in veterinary practice, and veterinary practice and public recognition and appreciation of VNs' extensive skills and knowledge base.

In summary

Empowering the VHCT and embracing different individual and professional perspectives at all stages of patient care is fundamental to the integration of nutritional assessment and the optimisation of nutritional care. Appropriate delegation and effective utilisation of all team members is needed to provide expert feeding advice and pet caretaker support in executing nutritional recommendations.

References

AAHA (American Animal Hospital Association) (2009a) *Compliance: Taking Quality Care to the Next Level: A Report of the 2009 AAHA Compliance Follow-up Study.* AAHA Press, Lakewood, Colorado.

AAHA (American Animal Hospital Association) (2009b) *Six Steps to Higher-quality Patient Care*. AAHA Press, Lakewood, Colorado.

AAHA (American Animal Hospital Association) (2010) Extended nutrition evaluations. Available at: https://www.aaha.org/globalassets/02-guidelines/nutritional-assessment/nutritionevaluationform.pdf (accessed 29 January 2022).

Abood, S.K. and Verton-Shaw, S. (2021) Talking about dog and cat nutrition with clients. *Veterinary Clinics of North America: Small Animal Practice*, 51 (3), 517–528.

Alvarez, E.E., Schultz, K.K., Floerchinger, A.M. and Hull, J.L. (2022) Small animal general practitioners discuss nutrition infrequently despite assertion of indication, citing barriers. *Journal of the American Veterinary Medical Association*, 260(13), 1704–1710.

AVMA (2022) Utilizing veterinary technicians to improve practice success. Available at: https://www.avma.org/resources-tools/practice-management/utilizing-veterinary-technicians-improve-practice-success (accessed 30 July 2022).

Blees, N.R., Vandendriessche, V.L., Corbee, R.J., Picavet, P. and Hesta, M. (2021) Nutritional consulting in regular veterinary practices in Belgium and the Netherlands. *Veterinary Medicine and Science*, 1–17.

Boatright, K. (2019) How to retain valued employees. *Today's Veterinary Practice*, 9(5), 94–96.

Boatright, K. (2021) The Most Underutilized Resource in Your Clinic. *Today's Veterinary Practice*, 11(1), 88–90.

Britton, A. (2019) A guide to successful veterinary nurse clinics: part 2. *VN Times*, 19(3). Available at: https://www.vettimes.co.uk/article/a-guide-to-successful-veterinary-nurse-clinics-part-2/ (accessed 16 February 2023).

Bruckner, I. and Handl, S. (2020) Survey on the role of nutrition in first-opinion practices in Austria and Germany: An evaluation of knowledge, preferences and need for further education. *Journal of Animal Physiology and Animal Nutrition*, 105 (Suppl. 2), 89–94.

Buzhardt, L. (2003) Implementing a feline preventive medicine program. Available at: https://www.dvm360.com/view/implementing-feline-preventive-medicine-program (accessed 3 August 2022).

Carter, H. and Grant, J. (2022) Turnover: Identifying causes and solutions. *Today's Veterinary Nurse*, 5(3), 10–13.

Chadwick, M. (2022) Rethinking the technician's role in the age of telemedicine. *Today's Veterinary Business*, 6(2), 6–7.

Chan, D.L. and Freeman, L.M. (2006). Nutrition in critical illness. *Veterinary Clinics of North America: Small Animal Practice*, 36, 1225–1241.

Cline, M.G., Burns, K.M., Coe, J.B., Downing, R., Durzi, T. *et al.* (2021) 2021 AAHA nutrition and weight management guidelines for dogs and cats. *Journal of the American Animal Hospital Association*, 57(4), 153–178.

Connolly, K.M., Heinze, C.R. and Freeman, L.M. (2014). Feeding practices of dog breeders in the United States and Canada. *Journal of the American Veterinary Medical Association*, 245(6), 669–676.

Corbee, R. J. (2019) Setting up a nurse-led nutrition service. *The Veterinary Nurse*. Available at: https://www.theveterinarynurse.com/review/article/setting-up-a-nurse-led-nutrition-service (accessed 16 February 2023).

Creevy, K.E., Grady, J., Little, S.E., Moore, G.E., Groetzinger Strickler, B. *et al.* (2019) 2019 AAHA canine life stage guidelines. *Journal of the American Animal Hospital Association*, 55(6), 267–290.

Donnelly, A. (2022) Trust the process. *Today's Veterinary Business*, 6(2), 64–65.

Du Marchie Sarvaas, C. (2022) Diagnostics can help profession keep pace with pet populations. *Veterinary Times,* 52(6), 10.

Fanning, J. and Shepherd, A.J. (2010) Contribution of veterinary technicians to veterinary business revenue. *Journal of the American Veterinary Medical Association,* 236(8), 846.

Freeman, L., Becvarova, I., Cave, N., MacKay, C., Nguyen, P. *et al.* (2011) WSAVA Nutritional assessment guidelines. *Journal of Small Animal Practice,* 52(7), 385–396.

Gerrard, E. (2015) Owner compliance – educating clients to act on pet care advice. *VN Times,* 15(4), 6–7.

Hancock, G. and Schubert, C. (2007) The utilisation of veterinary nurses in practice. *European Journal of Companion Animal Practice,* 17(2), 191–195.

Hollwarth, A. and Vickery, S. (2022) Nurse-led rabbit clinics. *The Veterinary Nurse.* Available at: https://www.theveterinarynurse.com/review/article/nurse-led-rabbit-clinics (accessed 16 February 2023).

Janke, N., Coe, J.B., Bernardo, T.M., Dewey, C.E. and Stone, E.A. (2021) Pet owners' and veterinarians' perceptions of information exchange and clinical decision-making in companion animal practice. *PLoS ONE,* 16(2), e0245632.

John, A. (2022) Protecting pets: how vet nurses can help educate owners. *VN Times,* 22(2), 12–14.

Johnson, L.N. and Linder, D. (2013) Making client communication appetising: talking with clients about nutrition. *The Veterinary Nurse,* 4(9), 542–548.

Kinnison, T. (2017) Portrayal of professions and occupations on veterinary practice websites and the potential for influencing public perceptions. *The Veterinary Nurse,* 8(10), 563–568.

Kinnison, T. and May, S.A. (2016) Evidence-based healthcare: The importance of effective interprofessional working for high quality veterinary services, a UK Example. *Veterinary Evidence.* Available at: http://dx.doi.org/10.18849/ve.v1i4.54 (accessed 6 February 2022).

Kinnison, T., May, S.A., Guile, D. (2014) Inter-professional practice: From veterinarian to the veterinary team. *Journal of Veterinary Medical Education,* 41, 172–178.

Kinnison, T., Guile, D., May, S.A. (2016) The case of veterinary interprofessional practice: From one health to a world of its own. *Journal of Interprofessional Education & Practice,* 4, 51–57

Lester, B. (2021) Let's embrace techs and tech. *Today's Veterinary Business,* 5(2), 34–37.

Little, G. (2013) Concordance and compliance. *In Focus.* Available at: https://www.veterinary-practice.com/article/concordance-and-compliance (accessed 3 August 2022).

Lumbis, R. and De Scally, M. (2020) Knowledge, attitudes and application of nutrition assessments by the veterinary health care team in small animal practice. *Journal of Small Animal Practice,* 61, 494–503.

Lynch, H. (2012) Developing a nutrition program in your practice. *Today's Veterinary Practice,* 2(4), 75–78.

McCormack, S. (2019) Companion animal nutrition: serious food for thought. *Veterinary Business Journal,* 193, 16–18.

Ograin, V.L. (2016) Implementing a nutritional consultation program in your hospital. Available at: https://www.isvma.org/wp-content/uploads/2016/10/IMPLEMENTINGANUTRITIONALCONSULTATIONPROGRAMINYOURHOSPITAL.pdf (accessed 3 August 2022).

Pet Nutrition Alliance (2018) Nutritional tools & resources for veterinary healthcare teams. Available at: https://petnutritionalliance.org/site/pnatool/our-practice-has-decided-to-implement-the-aaha-nutritional-assessment-guidelines-for-dogs-and-cats-how-can-we-introduce-the-concept-of-nutrition-as-the-fifth-vital-assessment-to-the-entire-veterinar-2/ (accessed 3 August 2022).

RCVS (Royal College of Veterinary Surgeons) (2022) Code of professional conduct for veterinary nurses. Available at: https://www.rcvs.org.uk/setting-standards/advice-and-guidance/code-of-professional-conduct-for-veterinary-nurses/ (accessed 28 July 2022).

Schleicher, M., Cash, S.B. and Freeman, L.M. (2019) Determinants of pet food purchasing decisions. *Canadian Veterinary Journal*, 60(6), 644–650.

Shock, D.A., Roche, S.M., Genore, R. and Renaud, D.L. (2020) The economic impact that registered veterinary technicians have on Ontario veterinary practices. *Canadian Veterinary Journal*, 61(5), 505–511.

Tassava, B. (2016) Establishing preventive care practice standards. *Veterinary Team Brief*, 4(4), 24–27.

Today's Veterinary Nurse (2022) Survey results shine light on pet owner perceptions of veterinary nurses. Available at: https://todaysveterinarynurse.com/veterinary-nurse-pet-owner-survey/ (accessed 1 August 2022).

Today's Veterinary Practice (2020) Conversation starters. Available at: https://mydigitalpublication.com/publication/?m=60565&i=672936&view=articleBrowser&article_id=3760690&search=Clinic%20Innovation%20Guide%20&ver=html5 (accessed 30 July 2022).

Verton-Shaw, S. (2016) *Promoting preventive nutrition. Veterinary Team Brief*, 4(4), 54–56.

Vet Times (2022) Transformational technology. *Vet Times*, 52(8), 18–20.

Veterinary Practice (2020) Should we be charging for nursing clinics? Available at: https://www.veterinary-practice.com/article/should-we-be-charging-for-nursing-clinics (accessed 28 July 2022).

Walsh, S. (2022) Leading by example. *Today's Veterinary Business*. 6(2), 58–69.

Ward, E. (2022) Consistency creates credibility. *Today's Veterinary Business*, 6(2), 14–17.

Wiggins, H. (2016) How to run a successful nurse clinic. *The Veterinary Nurse*, 7(5). Available at: https://www.theveterinarynurse.com/review/article/how-to-run-a-successful-nurse-clinic (accessed 16 February 2023).

Writer-Davies, S. (2019) The value of veterinary nurses to practice – changing the mind-set. Available at: https://www.vnfutures.org.uk/the-value-of-veterinary-nurses-to-practice-changing-the-mind-set/ (accessed 28 July 2022).

WSAVA (World Small Animal Veterinary Association) (2021) Global Nutrition Toolkit. Available at: https://wsava.org/wp-content/uploads/2021/04/WSAVA-Global-Nutrition-Toolkit-English.pdf (accessed 6 September 2022).

Yagi, K. (2017) What can veterinary nurses do for the practice? *Veterinary Team Brief*, 5(10), 21–25.

Yeates, J. (2014) The role of the veterinary nurse in animal welfare. *Veterinary Nursing Journal*, 29 (7), 250–251.

Applying theory to practice

9

Rachel Lumbis

Abstract

In this chapter, reference is made to patient scenarios that involve the provision of nutritional care using an interprofessional approach in a variety of clinical settings. These highlight how working as an interprofessional team can benefit different stakeholders including patients, clients, veterinary teams and veterinary practices, and offer appropriate reflection, evaluation and suggestions for future practice.

Please note these scenarios are not designed to provide detailed information of the nutritional care and support required or delivered in each case, however an overview of feeding management, nutritional risk factors and key requirements is provided where appropriate. All names have been changed and personal identifiable information removed to ensure anonymity. Thank you to the colleagues who have contributed to, and peer-reviewed, these scenarios.

Scenario 1: An African grey parrot with hypocalcaemia

Practice type: Exotics (first opinion)

The scenario

Bert, a 12-year-old, captive bred African grey parrot, *Psittacus erithacus,* (Fig. 9.1) is brought in by his caretakers following seizures, inappetence and general weakness at home. He has never been seen by a veterinarian so, on arrival at the veterinary practice, Bert is registered, and a brief history is taken by the receptionist, using the predetermined list of questions devised by the practice.

Bert was purchased as a hand-reared fledgling and was confirmed by the breeder to be male at the time of purchase. He is the sole bird in the house, and lives in a cage in the front room. A nutritional history revealed his diet consists of a sunflower seed-based diet, with occasional fruit and vegetables. He is also given human food, such as toast, crisps and biscuits as treats. For the past 12 hours, he has refused food and water and ceased communication with his caretakers.

© Rachel Lumbis and Tierney Kinnison 2023. *An Interprofessional Approach to Veterinary Nutrition* (R. Lumbis and T. Kinnison)
DOI: 10.1079/9781800621107.0009

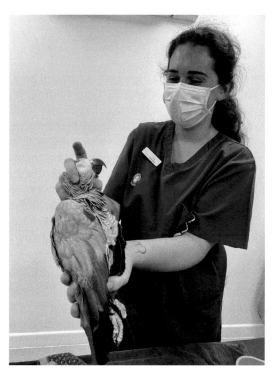

Fig. 9.1. A photo of Bert being held by one of the VNs during his visit to the veterinary practice. Photograph used with permission from Matthew Rendle.

A veterinarian is unavailable. One of the veterinary nurses (VNs), who has over 25 years of experience in the care and treatment of exotic pets and wildlife, refers to the receptionist's notes in the patient's clinical record, before inviting the caretakers to bring Bert through to a consult room for him to be triaged. Physical examination reveals neurological signs, including intermittent tonic seizures, and general weakness, with an inability to perch. Bert's body condition score (BCS) is 7/9 but his feathers are in poor condition and damaged.

The initial NA conducted by the receptionist highlights some risk factors, warranting an extended NA. These include:

- provision of an unbalanced diet and suboptimal environmental conditions
- history of inappetence and a refusal to consume food or water for the past 12 hours
- sedentary lifestyle.

Further questioning identifies that Bert is always indoors, with no access to UV light. It also reveals that the caretakers' employment circumstances have changed, and the husband now works entirely from home.

Communication

Between the VN and the caretaker

The caretakers ultimately just want their pet treated and back to good health ASAP. They see little value in the substantial questioning, first posed by the receptionist and then by the VN and become increasingly frustrated. The VN's extensive knowledge and experience of nursing patients with a similar presentation influences their line of questioning, making this critical to obtaining a relevant and comprehensive history. It also ensures that that the veterinarian is fully informed, thus facilitating an accurate diagnosis and the rapid instigation of treatment. The caretakers' lack of knowledge is a challenge; they are adamant that Bert is being housed in optimal conditions and are convinced of his 'male' gender. However, from the history and physical examination, the VN suspects that poor diet and husbandry have contributed to Bert's symptoms.

Between the VN and the veterinarian

The veterinarian involved with this patient has limited experience of African grey parrots and has never seen one presenting in this way. In contrast, the VN has seen numerous birds present like this over many years and has to relay to the veterinarian a few key points.

- Taking radiographs and a blood sample from this species is quick and straightforward.
- Despite the display of neurological signs, this will not automatically elevate Bert's anaesthetic risk to a level that will mean that performing diagnostics under anaesthetic will be considered unsafe.
- The signalment of this case highlights the potential for the following commonalities:
  - o a seed-based diet is completely unsuitable for this (and any) parrot species, therefore Bert has likely been malnourished all his life
  - o African grey parrots require UVB light in captivity
  - o 'Bert' has been incorrectly sexed and is almost certainly female
  - o the cause of Bert's clinical signs is likely acute hypocalcaemia, secondary to folliculogenesis which has occurred because of the male caregiver, with whom the bird is bonded and who now works from home and is therefore close to Bert for extended periods of time.
- Patients usually respond quickly to a combination of oral and injectable calcium, combined with oral tube feeding, followed by a complete change of diet and husbandry including the daily provision of UVB light.

Between the VN and the veterinary healthcare team

People can be fearful of birds for many reasons, including a fear of getting bitten or scratched and a fear of them dying under anaesthetic. Following Bert's admission, the VN communicates with the team to provide appropriate reassurance and identifies members of the team for whom further training and practice in handling will be beneficial.

Trust and value

In this scenario, the role of the receptionist, VN and veterinarian are valued, and team efficiency is maximised with full utilisation of the VN's skills and knowledge base. Mutual trust between all roles is also demonstrated, which is especially important for the veterinarian and VN. The veterinarian trusts the VN and welcomes their professional viewpoint, suggestions regarding patient care and treatment, and guidance and support in conducting the necessary diagnostic tests, helping to ensure a rapid diagnosis and provision of appropriate care and treatment. The VN is more experienced and knowledgeable on the care of this species, yet respects the role and responsibilities of the veterinarian and works in accordance with the UK's RCVS code conduct for VNs, fulfilling their professional responsibilities and maintaining the five principles of practice (RCVS, 2022):

1. Professional competence.
2. Honesty and integrity.
3. Independence and impartiality.
4. Client confidentiality and trust.
5. Professional accountability.

Professional roles and responsibilities

As the front of house, receptionists and client care staff are often the first team members to interact with clients. As such, together with the main appearance of the practice, the welcome provided by these individuals can heavily influence a client's first impressions of a practice. The receptionist provides a warm and professional welcome and establishes rapport with Bert's caretakers while asking relevant questions about his medical history, helping to create a positive first impression. The VN gathers further vital information, continues building trust, takes Bert's history and shares this information with the veterinarian before assisting with necessary diagnostic and medical treatment. The veterinarian considers all the acquired information and makes a diagnosis, leading the treatment plan. This example of a synergistic relationship between team members can optimise clinical output and, perhaps most importantly, animal welfare, and should therefore be a key goal of interprofessional practice and culture.

The veterinarian feels out of their clinical comfort zone and therefore under significant pressure. Working alongside a VN who has seen many patients present with a similar signalment and who has many years of experience in the handling, care and treatment of exotic pets is considered a great asset. Such mutual respect fosters team members' ability to support one another, step in when needed, and take account of others' duties (Hunter and Shaw, 2015). Yet some veterinarians are reluctant to take clinical guidance from VNs and this can be a challenge and a potential limitation. Lessons can be learnt if honesty and integrity are maintained and if concerns or deficits in clinical knowledge, skills, confidence and competence are shared with colleagues in a non-judgemental and blame-free environment.

Reflection and evaluation

Nutritional support and advice should be sought from the team member with the most expertise, knowledge and skills, not necessarily according to status or role. Yet, it is essential to be conscious of, and work according to, one's own level of competence and confidence. The positive team approach in this scenario results in the patient being seen quickly and an accurate history being obtained. This ensures the provision of a rapid and accurate diagnosis and timely implementation of the necessary care and treatment, ultimately benefiting the patient and representing good welfare standards. Client experience is also positive and showcases the roles and responsibilities of the veterinary healthcare team (VHCT).

Suggestions for future practice

For common clinical scenarios such as this one, the provision of a written care bundle consisting of relevant information to help inform and guide each stage of patient care and treatment could prove valuable for all members of the VHCT.

Scenario 2: A horse admitted as a medical colic

Practice type: Equine (referral)

The scenario

Ludovic (Ludo) was admitted as a medical colic. After a full physical examination, the veterinarian suspects chronic grass sickness (EGS, or equine dysautonomia). A definitive cause of grass sickness is unknown but involves damage to the nervous system, the main symptom being intestinal dysmotility (Pirie and McGorum *et al.*, 2018). It can be acute, sub-acute and chronic. Clinical signs of the chronic form progress slowly and include profound cachexia, generalised myasthenia, tachycardia and mild signs of gastrointestinal dysfunction (Lavoie, 2020). Horses suffering from the chronic form become depressed and anorexic, quickly resulting in weight loss and emaciation. Prognosis is guarded, but with nutritional support, time and intense veterinary nursing care, chronic cases can recover.

Communication

In equine cases, nutritional support frequently involves calculations and the science of nutrition, which is often led by veterinarians. However, in this case, these factors were less significant as Ludo refused to eat. Subsequently, whole team involvement became necessary, with a lot of the care being delegated by veterinarians to the VNs and patient care assistants. Communication was therefore very important and involved accurate record-keeping, including the provision of a clear and current log of what feed the horse had been offered each day, how much had been eaten and daily recording of body weight. This information, together with an evaluation of Ludo's progress was discussed daily among the team and regularly reported back to the owner.

Patients with chronic conditions such as this can be hospitalised for months, putting great strain on communication. The hospital uses a paper-based filing system so Ludo's file needs to be kept in order and the reception team have responsibility for the regular scanning of paperwork to avoid it getting lost or damaged.

Over the course of his hospitalisation, team members develop increasing interest in and emotional attachment to Ludo. Yet data protection and client confidentiality still have to be maintained and all staff are vigilant to avoid discussing the patient outside of work and with other clients.

Trust and value

As Ludo is anorexic, determining what food would entice spontaneous food intake is a priority. From a care perspective, this patient scenario provides the opportunity for the VNs and technicians to take the lead as nutritional support is fundamental to recovery. The veterinarians consider their colleague's knowledge and experience of different feed products to be superior to their own and trust them to source the appropriate feed, record what had been offered and communicate the outcome. Between them, the VNs and technicians also have greater opportunity to spend time and build up a relationship with Ludo, thus increasing the likelihood of food intake. This is a great strength in the team, and it also allows for a good relationship to be established with the horse's caretaker as they see how hard the team are working together. Where further knowledge and expertise is required, an external nutritional advisor is consulted. This understanding and appreciation of professional roles helps to encourage appropriate empowerment of VNs and support staff, overcome time as a limiting factor and promote confidence in the VHCT's provision of nutritional advice and support.

Professional roles and responsibilities

In this scenario, the veterinarians follow the medical model of healthcare, with primary emphasis on the treatment of disease and relief of symptoms. The VNs and technicians follow a more holistic approach and spend, in comparison, significantly more time with Ludo and his caretaker, becoming more emotionally involved which, at times, clouds judgements. This is not to say the veterinarians are not emotionally involved, but their focus on the disease process facilitates a more pragmatic approach to patient treatment and care.

On occasions, professional responsibilities can conflict with each other, presenting a dilemma and need for veterinary professionals to balance their professional responsibilities while having a primary regard for animal welfare (RCVS, 2022). This scenario prompts frequent discussions surrounding patient welfare. With the involvement of multiple team members and representation across different roles, opinions regarding ongoing patient care and treatment were varied and emotions became fraught. The receptionists and support staff raised concerns over the welfare and ethics of continuing care. After several weeks of hospitalisation, even the VNs questioned the decision to continue care rather than opt for euthanasia, presenting the challenge of continued involvement with the case while contradicting one's own ethical viewpoint. Maintaining interprofessional trust and respect, while maintaining awareness of personal role and responsibilities is very important and results in a good outcome in this case.

Reflection and evaluation

In this scenario, teamwork and effective collaboration is paramount to success. Every member of the VHCT plays a vital role and their involvement is valued. At the twice daily ward rounds, representatives from the teams of veterinarians, VNs and technicians are present and contribute equally to discussions. No one's knowledge on the 'art' of nutrition is considered stronger than the others.

Team interrelations are enhanced by building mutual trust in, and respect for, each other's skills and knowledge. Veterinarians' recognition and appropriate utilisation of colleagues is demonstrated, with VNs and technicians actively involved in the discussion of the patient's care and treatment and able to showcase their knowledge, skills and overall competence. This promotes veterinarians' confidence in their ability, thus enabling them to concentrate on the work that only they are qualified to perform. Yet the scenario highlights the importance of being aware and accepting of any knowledge or skill deficits and seeking external advice when required. The opportunity to learn from the expert advice and professional opinion of an external equine nutritionist is fully embraced.

At times, the welfare and ethics of continuing patient care is questioned by the VNs and technicians, as well as support staff, which, ultimately, strengthens their respect for and trust in the veterinarians' knowledge. This enhanced teamwork results in better patient care and the provision of a professional service to clients, with excellent care and communication. The team's efficiency also benefits the practice by contributing to a positive reputation, enabling more patients to be treated, with improved profit margins.

Suggestions for future practice

Along with intense feelings of responsibility, emotional investment in Ludo's health and wellbeing is high, particularly among the VNs and veterinary technicians, leading to a risk of emotional fatigue. Affected horses can be hospitalised for several weeks and are often dull and depressed. Staff morale can be quickly lost, and the uncertainty of the outcome is always a concern. Colleagues demonstrate support for one another, and senior management ensure that team members have opportunities to debrief and discuss personal feelings openly and honestly, without judgement. Further support is also available to student and qualified veterinary professionals, and non-clinical staff, through Vetlife and the RCVS Mind Matters Initiative (MMI) and this would be better highlighted to staff in the future.

Scenario 3: A guinea pig with malocclusion

Practice type: Small animal (charity)

The scenario

Sage, a female Abyssinian guinea pig (*Cavia porcellus*) is presented for a weight check due to a reduction in appetite. The caretaker doesn't have the funds to pay for a veterinary consultation, so the receptionist offers a complimentary appointment with one of the VNs. The VN weighs Sage and asks the caretaker for permission to perform a physical examination, including a nutritional assessment (NA). It is Sage's first visit to the veterinary practice so no previous medical history is available. Her caretaker estimates her to be around 2 years. Sage's bodyweight is 0.58 kg and her BCS is 2/5 (thin). Her ribs, hips and spine are all easily palpable with no pressure and some abdominal curving is evident. Given the lack of medical history, there are no previous measurements for comparison but from these findings, the VN estimates that Sage is between 10–20% below her ideal body weight (PFMA, 2015). Oral examination is difficult due to Sage's small mouth but the VN visualises incisor elongation and an inability to fully close her mouth. There is also evidence of excessive salivation. One of the student VNs assists the qualified VN during the consultation by asking relevant questions and obtaining a thorough husbandry and nutritional history.

Several additional nutritional risk factors are identified. A commercial guinea pig muesli-style (mixed ration) diet contributes to the majority of Sage's daily food intake. As selective feeders, guinea pigs typically select the most palatable food items, resulting in imbalanced nutrition. Further risk factors include a lack of regular provision of fresh food, grass, hay and vitamin C supplementation, and the daily provision of treats including dried fruit and yogurt drops. Sage's clinical record is updated accordingly with details of her physical examination and NA. The nutritional risk factors are highlighted to the caretaker who is commended for identifying Sage's ill health and for seeking veterinary treatment. The VN's findings are discussed with one of the veterinarians who recommends a full veterinary consultation and examination, with further treatment to be carried out as required. Cost is a significant concern for the caretaker who doesn't qualify for free service but who is eligible for low-cost service. The practice manager arranges a payment plan for veterinary treatment.

Veterinary examination confirms a need for oral examination and radiography under general anaesthesia. Oral examination reveals overgrowth and misalignment of the premolars and molars, confirmed by radiographic imaging (Fig. 9.2), with subsequent overgrowth of the incisors and entrapment of the tongue. A dental is performed.

Under direct supervision of a qualified VN, the discharge appointment is conducted by the student VN who explains about the aetiology of malocclusion. Due to guinea pigs' open-rooted elodont teeth, a nutritional recommendation is given to feed a diet that promotes natural dental wear, meets Sage's nutritional requirements and which provides appropriate environmental enrichment:

- Stop feeding the muesli-style diet and colourful guinea pig treats available in many pet stores. These can be high in sugar, low in fibre and can contribute to selective feeding, dental and gastrointestinal disease and obesity. Replace with a diet consisting of grass-based pellets, offering no more than 15 g a day. Processed food has a soft consistency and insufficiently abrasive texture, resulting in limited chewing and poor dental wear, with subsequent dental elongation and malocclusion.
- Supply unlimited good quality hay and fresh grass, both of which are an essential form of fibrous and low-calorie food and promote natural dental wear.
- Ensure the provision of 10–30 mg/kg vitamin C per day, depending on physiologic state.

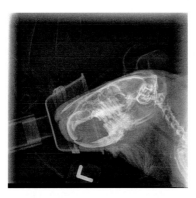

Fig. 9.2. Left lateral radiograph of a guinea pig skull revealing overgrown premolar and molar teeth. Author's own image.

- Offer food items rich in vitamin C such as broccoli, cabbage and parsley. A list is provided.
- Treats should be limited to guinea-pig safe fresh fruit, given in small amounts occasionally due to their high sugar content and contribution to weight gain. Instead, the caretaker is advised to provide sources of environmental enrichment in place of edible treats, such as tunnels and hides. Details of guinea pig-friendly fruit are provided.
- Guinea pigs develop their dietary preferences and imprint on food items early in life and later changes to food provision or management can result in food refusal (Quesenberry and Carpenter, 2012), underpinning the need for regular monitoring and support post hospitalisation.

A personalised husbandry and nutritional recommendation is communicated to the caregiver verbally and via email, as well as being documented in Sage's clinical record. A generic guinea-pig care sheet is also provided in hard and electronic copy. A receptionist provides a sample bag of high-quality hay and a grass-based pellet diet, labelled with the correct amount to be fed per day, and associated product information. Details of the follow-up appointment are supplied in person and via email.

Two days later, the student VN performs a follow-up phone call to the caretaker enquiring about Sage and to see how she is getting on with the new diet. Sage likes the pellets and hay, but the caretaker is reluctant to purchase more from the veterinary practice due to the cost. The student empathises but reiterates how diet is the determining factor for development of dental disease in guinea pigs and explains how alternative, cheaper products are not always suitable. Appropriate diets are outlined to the client, together with a reminder about the positive effect that the recommended diet has on quality and length of life, disease prevention and potential future cost of veterinary care. The caretaker is praised for supplementing the diet with fresh foods to help provide Sage with adequate fibre, moisture and enrichment.

A week later, Sage returns for a post-op check with the veterinarian who performed the dental surgery. The husbandry and nutritional recommendation is reiterated, together with the importance of adherence for the long-term maintenance of Sage's health and wellbeing and prevention of future dental disease. The veterinarian updates Sage's clinical records, including a current body weight and condition score, and adds her details to the diary for a follow-up phone call with a receptionist in a month's time.

Communication

When seeing a patient for the first time, there is a lot to ask, examine and assess to get a comprehensive overview of the patient's condition and caretaker's values and preferences. Effective communication between the qualified VN, student VN and caretaker is fundamental to developing a positive connection and a reliable and trustful relationship with the client. It is also crucial to establishing the VHCT as a vital part of the relationship between pet and caretaker, thus enhancing the human–animal bond (HAB). Utilising the skills of VNs to collect information prior to consultation with a veterinarian and to provide other specific VN-led services can have several benefits. These include the provision of more time and cost-effective practice, enabling veterinarians to focus on the completion of tasks only they are qualified to complete, and enhancement of the profile of the VN role among the general public.

Appropriate liaison and communication is maintained between other team members involved in the care of the patient, with appropriate referral where required. When both a VN and veterinarian communicate with clients, caretakers are more involved in decision-making regarding their pet's healthcare (Janke *et al.*, 2022). Furthermore, VNs' communication can significantly enhance client engagement in decision-making when working collaboratively with veterinarians. Providing consistency between team members and a 'one voice' approach to veterinary treatment and nutritional care and support helps to create credibility. At all stages of Sage's care, appropriate levels of information are provided, together with a summary of what is said to help facilitate understanding. Caretakers essentially want the best possible care for their pets and, while financial limitations can influence the dietary decision-making process, the provision of clear, reliable and regular communication helps to ensure compliance and concordance.

Trust and value

In this scenario, the client's finances are limited and the initial VN consultation is provided free of charge. While this results in rapid treatment provision and a positive patient outcome, an enhanced client experience and increased practice productivity, the VN's contribution to the generated revenue is hidden in the cost of services and procedures. 'Free' has no perceived value and so ensuring greater transparency of the work completed by VNs enables clearer revelation of VN-related revenue and an associated appreciation. Given that veterinarians' consultation time is charged for in addition to services, some might suggest the potential missed opportunity to charge appropriately for a VN's time, skills and knowledge. An associated charge can offer direct contribution to practice revenue, promote greater client trust, respect and compliance with recommendations, empower VNs with autonomy and with feelings of being better valued as professionals. However, on this occasion, the initial VN consultation showcases the proficiency, role and responsibility of the VN and enables the client to seek expert advice.

Sage is placed at the centre of the veterinary and nutritional recommendations, and a clear explanation is given to the caretaker regarding how and why these will benefit her health and wellbeing. Expectations are also clearly communicated to help reduce the chances of future dental disease. When recommending and selling pet food, clients can question the VHCT's financial motivations, believing that promotion of a particular brand may result in their personal gain. Providing suggestions of appropriate types of pet food, including details of brands (if requested) can help to reduce concerns behind the nutrition recommendations being made and enable an informed decision to be made by the client (Janke *et al.*, 2021). The higher the pet–caretaker and vet–client bond, the higher the level of care expected, meaning an increased likelihood of recommendations being followed, regardless of cost (Lue *et al.*, 2008). Providing an overview of the veterinary services' value, a clear rationale behind the recommendations being made and ensuring the caretaker's understanding of and concordance with this further helps to build trust, acceptance, perception of value and a willingness to pay for the necessary veterinary care and treatment.

Where possible, the client is paired with the same members of the VHCT to help ensure continuity and establish a personal, rather than transactional, relationship. Continuity helps to build a bond between veterinary professional, caretaker and pet, resulting in a higher likelihood of a trusting relationship. Subsequently, caretakers' acceptance of recommendations and compliance is more likely, as is their endorsement of the veterinary practice to friends, family members and colleagues.

Professional roles and responsibilities

The acquisition and interpretation of a husbandry and nutritional history is an excellent way to utilise motivated and knowledgeable VNs, students, patient care assistants and reception staff (Miller, 2022). It also provides an invaluable source of information, particularly in exotic pet species for whom suboptimal diet and husbandry is a key contributor to ill health and disease. In this scenario, a qualified VN supervises a student VN in taking a history and asking relevant questions. Providing appropriate training, mentoring and interprofessional support can help to produce a VHCT whose members are competent and confident in recognising which details are important to elaborate on, which is a valuable asset to the veterinary team and practice (Miller, 2022).

The provision of a clinical diagnosis and prognosis is considered beyond the legal scope of the VN's role and is limited to veterinarians. Yet through the accurate identification of a number of nutritional risk factors, the VN suspects that a lack of fibrous roughage is contributing to dental disease which ultimately results in the timely provision of appropriate treatment. The veterinarian is accepting and supportive of the VN's concerns and reiterates these to the caretaker.

Financial constraints are a reality of veterinary practice and it is essential for the VHCT to work within clients' financial means to fulfil their professional, ethical and legal obligations and responsibilities to patients (Boatright, 2020). In this situation, the practice manager is instrumental to minimising financial barriers and considering deals that could make optimal nutrition more affordable, for example, buy two dietary products get one half price.

Reflection and evaluation

Incorrect and inadequate husbandry and feeding practices are a leading cause of illness in exotic animal pets, with many diseases linked to, or caused by, incorrect nutrition, therefore obtaining a thorough history is a cornerstone of exotic pet medicine.

Empowerment of the VHCT is fundamental to the integration of NA and the optimisation of nutritional care. Appropriate delegation and effective utilisation of all team members enables the provision expert feeding advice and pet caretaker support in executing nutritional recommendations. Clear communication of expectations and value, together with effective interprofessional teamwork, and high quality care, treatment and service provision further helps to ensure client satisfaction and subsequent promotion of the veterinary practice and team to others. Provided adequate training, practice support and colleague referral is given, offering VN consultations, as well as VN (topic-specific) clinics can help to demonstrate that veterinary professionals can provide more than clinical support. It can also help to prevent clients from seeking preventative healthcare and associated advice from elsewhere.

Scenario 4: Feline obesity

Practice type: Small animal (first opinion)

The scenario

Tabitha, an 11-year-old, 8.1 kg neutered female domestic shorthair cat presents at the practice for a veterinary examination following a fight with another cat. Her BCS is estimated to be 8/9 (WSAVA, 2023). Muscle mass is normal.

Following admission and treatment of injuries, the veterinarian calls Tabitha's caretaker to provide an update and arrange collection from the hospital. The caretaker is informed that Tabitha is carrying excess weight and, following a brief discussion about the risks associated with obesity, is advised that she would benefit from some dietary modification. At discharge, this information is verbally reiterated by a VN and supplemented with written information about feline obesity and ways to increase activity levels in cats. Due to a lack of available consultation rooms, the discharge appointment is conducted in the waiting room. Rather than enter into a potentially sensitive conversation regarding weight management in public, the VN asks the caretaker if they would like to arrange an appointment with the practice's nutrition champion for a more in-depth discussion and NA. The caretaker is reluctant to bring Tabitha into the practice again so soon but agrees when advised it can be combined with her post-op check. A receptionist schedules the appointment for ten days' time and provides an electronic copy of a nutritional history form for the caretaker to complete at home and submit to the practice prior to this. The caretaker agrees to receiving appointment reminders and relevant associated information via text and email.

A follow-up email, together with a link to the nutritional history form is sent a few days later, reminding the caretaker to complete and return the form. The practice's contact number and an email address is provided in case of any queries regarding the form. The day before the visit, a courtesy call is made by a member of the reception team, thanking the caretaker for submitting the form and providing a reminder about Tabitha's appointment the following day.

Tabitha returns for an appointment with the practice's nutrition champion, a VN. The post-op check is performed first then, having read Tabitha's notes and reviewed her nutritional history form beforehand, the VN asks for permission to discuss her diet and weight. At previous preventative healthcare appointments, no comments had been made by the veterinarian regarding Tabitha's weight and BCS, therefore the caretaker believed that Tabitha was an optimal body condition and ideal weight, and just 'a chunky cat'. The VN is empathetic and listens before asking what diet is being fed and why. Tabitha is fed a commercial diet designed for adult cats and receives canned food three times a day, coinciding with the owner's meal times. She also has access to dry food throughout the day to encourage normal feeding behaviour. The care-taker uses treat provision, including human foods such as cream cheese and milk, as a way of expressing their love for Tabitha and for rewarding her good behaviour, all of which constitute more than 10% of her total daily calorie intake. She chooses to spend limited time outside but is known to be a suc-cessful hunter (Fig. 9.3). An NA is completed, including a demonstration of how to perform a BCS and associated discussion. Although disappointed, the client appears to agree with the score and acknowledges the identified nutri-tional risk factors and risks associated with obesity, demonstrating concern for Tabitha's health and wellbeing. Through this, the VN determines the client

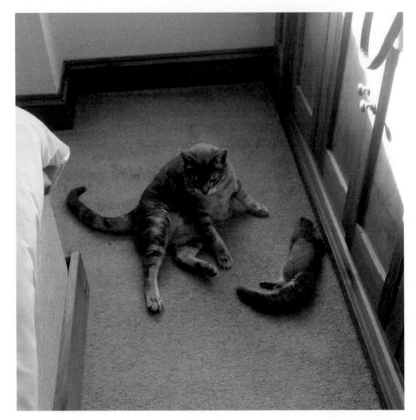

Fig. 9.3. 'Hunter' cats may kill prey due to their natural instinctive behaviour as opposed to hunger, however it is important to consider this potential food source, alongside others, such as well-meaning neighbours. Photograph: author.

as being ready for change. Goals and expectations are discussed and agreed with the caretaker and a detailed verbal and written nutritional recommendation is provided. This includes a feeding plan, including recommendations relating to the provision of treats and other supplementary food; details of recommended diets, reasons for this recommendation and how they will help Tabitha; instructions for diet transitioning; and details of available pet weight loss support, including enrolment onto the practice's weight management programme. This information is also sent to the caretaker via email. The VN also takes photographs of Tabitha to help visualise future weight loss (or gain) and checks the caretaker's understanding, offering the opportunity to ask any questions.

Before leaving the practice, a receptionist provides the caretaker with a sample bag of a weight loss prescription diet with a product brochure on how it works and written instructions of how much to feed at each meal. The caretaker is also informed about the time, costs, benefits and limitations of the practice's weight management programme. A follow-up appointment is made for a month's time with the nutrition champion at the weight management clinic. This is detailed on a business card and also emailed to the client. The caretaker is asked if they have any questions or queries before leaving the practice.

A follow-up courtesy call is made by a member of the reception team a week later to enquire about the dietary transition, to help clarify any queries and to provide a reminder of Tabitha's next appointment. When asked if Tabitha likes the weight management diet, the caretaker responds positively but feels it isn't working as Tabitha weighs the same and, after hearing from a pet shop worker that veterinarians receive commission for product sales, declines the opportunity to purchase a bag from the practice. The myth is dispelled and the receptionist leverages the human–animal bond, reiterating the VHCT's desire and priority to support the owner in optimising Tabitha's health, welfare, wellbeing, quality of life and longevity. The caretaker is referred back to the details of recommended diets, restating the reasons for this recommendation and how they will help Tabitha. A recommendation is also given to switch to a smaller food bowl to accommodate the caretakers' tendency to offer a full bowl of food (Davies, 2022). The caregiver is also reminded that weight loss is a steady process, requiring dedication and ongoing support. The receptionist updates Tabitha's clinical record and asks the nutrition champion to call the caretaker to discuss any challenges to weight loss and to help identify potential solutions before the next appointment.

Communication

Obesity is a multifactorial disorder, and the multitude of underlying causes creates for a potentially challenging conversation with clients, necessitating a team approach. Like many veterinary scenarios, communication, understanding and adherence is key. Caretakers may experience feelings including shock, denial and guilt when obesity is first diagnosed and may perceive weight loss programmes as a threat to their bond with their pet, therefore initiation of the topic should be centred on the health and wellbeing of the pet. Here, the nutrition champion followed a modified '5 As' model to promote behaviour change (Hodgkiss *et al.*, 2020). Initially, the caretaker was 'asked' for permission to discuss Tabitha's diet and weight, before entering a cyclical process of performing a nutritional 'assessment', 'advising' about the risks associated with obesity, 'agreeing' the goals and expectations and 'assisting' through support provision. Despite education of the secondary diseases and reduction in quality of life and life expectancy that result from obesity, caretakers may not always be willing to follow a nutritional recommendation or be ready to make a commitment to change their pet's diet. Determining a client's readiness for change and accepting this can help to reduce VHCT anxiety and frustration around nutrition conversations (Mattson, 2021). In this situation, the caretaker initially appeared ready to implement change, but many are not. The following points outline a potential course of action in two different scenarios:

1. The client hasn't acknowledged or come to terms with their pet being classed as overweight or obese.
- It is too soon to prescribe and implement an action plan.
- Demonstrate concern for the pet's body weight and condition.
- Advise that the pet returns in a month's time for a weight check, ideally with the practice's nutrition champion, or with a VN or a motivated and trained patient care assistant. This encourages the client to return to the veterinary practice and reinforces the VHCT as the primary and trusted source of pet care and nutrition advice.
- Ensure that the pet's clinical records are updated to include the advice and nutritional recommendation given. Body weight and condition must be recorded on the patient's clinical notes, so future changes can be monitored.

2. The client is aware of their pet's weight gain but doesn't appear ready to take action.
- It is too soon to prescribe and implement an action plan.
- Try and help to identify challenges to weight loss and offer potential solutions.
- Reiterate that the VHCT is available to provide help and support as and when the caretaker is ready to discuss the matter further.

Caregivers who understand the detrimental impact of being overweight and who embrace the concept of lifelong weight control through diet and exercise are more likely to maintain an optimal bodyweight and condition for their pet (Davies, 2022). Successful communication requires consistency and reinforcement from all members of the VHCT (Ward, 2022a). Although usually only one member of the VHCT is in consultation with a client at a time, communication is a collective competence, requiring the consideration of systems and teams rather than individuals. The use of various communication strategies and support mechanisms can enable the VHCT to explore each client's unique relationship with their pet while preserving the bond between caretaker and pet (Linder, 2021).

Trust and value

Food provision is considered a primary means of expressing care and so the VHCT should focus their diet-related marketing and nutrition conversations on the bond between caretaker, pet and VHCT. Effective communication builds trust, and with trust it is possible to discuss challenging cases with more tolerance and understanding. In scenarios such as this, obtaining a comprehensive nutritional history provides not only an insight into the diet being consumed, but also an indication of the caretaker's beliefs, preferences and priorities, and their relationship with their pet. For example, Tabitha's caretaker considered treat provision to be a fundamental expression of love for their pet and believed that facilitating normal feeding behaviour was an important part of feeding management. Consideration of such viewpoints is integral to creating an individualised weight loss plan and not only increases overall chances of success, but also strengthens the bond between pet, caretaker, VHCT and practice (Linder, 2021; Johnson, 2022). Providing continuity in the VHCT members seen at each visit, and in the consistency of advice given and protocols followed, further helps to improve caretaker's trust in the VHCT and compliance with recommendations.

Clients don't always have to purchase a diet to get value from a nutritional conversation and consultation with the VHCT. In this scenario, the client was given physical items to help create a connection with the nutritional recommendation being given. These included:

- A hard and electronic copy of the nutritional recommendation, including suitable diet choices. The provision of dietary options helps to reduce clients' concerns behind the VHCT's motivations for recommending and selling pet food and enables them to make an informed decision (Janke *et al.*, 2021).
- A sample of an appropriate weight management diet, together with product information outlining its key nutritional factors.

An appropriately sized measuring cup that can be filled for each meal is another example of a physical item that could be given. These can be a useful aid, especially for clients who are new to a pet weight loss programme, however they are imprecise, particularly in situations like these when even a slight increase in food intake can be detrimental to the desired outcome.

Professional roles and responsibilities

Obesity is a modern-day epidemic in both people and companion animals. Veterinarians have an ethical and professional obligation to discuss and diagnose overweight and obesity in small animal practice (Kipperman and German, 2018). Yet every team member assumes an important role in making a diagnosis and in the delivery of patient care and treatment. In this scenario, no previous comments had been made in the patient's clinical record by a veterinary professional regarding Tabitha's weight and BCS. Potential reasons for this include short consult times, concerns over causing offence and not wanting to enter into a potentially controversial conversation or lengthy debate. However, discussion and documentation of nutrition, diet and exercise should be included in every standard patient examination, regardless of whether or not body weight and condition are considered an issue (Freeman *et al.*, 2011). Without a record, it is impossible to objectively assess changes over time or accurately educate clients, making conversations with caretakers even more challenging. Effective use of the VHCT can help to overcome potential barriers

and assist veterinarians in fulfilling this obligation and providing recommendations to prevent and address overweight and obesity in companion animals.

In this scenario, following the diagnosis of obesity, referral was made to
the most appropriate team member, whether that be a VN, nutrition champion,
receptionist/client service personnel or veterinarian. At the initial discharge
appointment, the VN realised that the busy waiting area was not an ideal or
safe environment for a discussion about obesity and instead arranged for a
private consultation with the practice's nutrition champion. Not all practices
have the luxury of appointing a dedicated nutrition champion, and not all VNs
are sufficiently comfortable or confident to conduct a VN-led consultation or
clinic. It is therefore important to play to the team's strengths and be open and
honest about individual differences – for example, identifying an individual's
strengths, aspects of the role they most and least enjoy, and aspects they
consider to be most difficult and challenging. Responsibility should be allo-
cated based on individual strengths and be within the individual's personal
and professional limits, with the provision of interprofessional support and
further training where required. Every team member should feel part of the
team and feel they have an influential impact. Engaged employees enjoy their
work more which is good for the professional wellness of the practice as well as
for clients and the health and welfare of patients.

The nutrition champion led the weight management consultations with
the caretaker and performed NAs on Tabitha yet, together with collaboration
from colleagues, was jointly responsible for:

- weighing the pet and then calculating weight loss at follow-up visits
- assisting the veterinarian by recording a nutritional history, evaluating
  the pet's current diet and explaining why this is unfavourable, and developing appropriate nutritional recommendations, including the provision
  of a nutritional plan to optimise body condition
- educating the caretaker on the pet health benefits of maintaining a lean
  body weight and communicating the nutritional recommendation and plan
- working with support staff to perform follow-up calls and appointments
  to support the caretaker in executing nutritional recommendations and
  facilitate owner compliance
- checking progress with weight loss and condition on a regular basis (at
  least monthly)
- providing support, encouragement and motivation to the client to adhere
  to the nutrition recommendation and weight management programme,
  and rewarding them (and the pet) when progress is made.

While not specifically outlined in this scenario, the role of a practice manager,
supervisor or team leader is also often integral to patient weight management
through the following responsibilities:

- Overseeing the creation of a task force (including at least one person from
  each role represented in the practice team) to build a weight management

programme. Determining the timeline for implementation of the programme, supporting the task force, holding members accountable for deadlines, assisting with logistical and budgetary needs, and making sure all critical decisions and topics are addressed (Troyer and Goodman Lee, 2013).

- Implementing and supervising practice protocols. Ensuring these are distributed to every team member.
- Liaising with the entire practice team to ensure the organisation of appropriate education of clients and the VHCT. Because of the potential for difficult client conversations, training for role-playing and verbal communication skill-building may be required (Troyer and Goodman Lee, 2013).
- Collaborating with veterinary professionals in the practice to establish a physical rehabilitation programme and/or referral system for exercise in obese patients.

Given the difficulty in achieving body weight and fat loss, caretakers can quickly become demotivated and sceptical if limited or no progress is made. Once concerns have been identified and discussed, it is important for team members to provide ongoing motivation, support and positive reinforcement, even if clients are reluctant to engage, and to reiterate the VHCT as the primary and trusted source of nutrition advice. Proactive team members will review the pet's clinical records, identify any previous dietary recommendations made by the veterinarian or VN and highlight/discuss these with the caretaker to get an update on compliance. Showcasing pets that have successfully achieved or maintained their target weight, and their caretakers' success stories, can further help to maintain client enthusiasm and commitment.

Reflection and evaluation

Obesity is considered the second most common health problem in pet cats in developed countries. Factors which significantly increase a cat's risk of obesity occur early on in life, before adulthood is reached (Rowe *et al.*, 2017), therefore focus should be placed on client education and prevention rather than reversal. Normalising communication regarding a pet's diet, weight status and the health risks associated with obesity can also help to support greater caretaker awareness and the establishment of a weight management partnership between client and the VHCT (Wainwright *et al.*, 2022). Yet time during veterinary consultations is limited and, while many clients would like, and benefit from, the provision of nutritional advice at veterinary appointments, priority is placed on addressing the primary reasons for their pet's visit to the clinic. Hence the need for entire team involvement and effort.

Obesity is a complex nutritional disorder that is challenging for the VHCT and pet caretakers to address and manage. Failure to comply with veterinary recommendations is the principal reason why caretakers lose control of their pet's body condition (Porsani *et al.*, 2020). In this scenario, the practice and VHCT employed a number of good habits which, together, can contribute to greater chances of compliance (AAHA, 2009) and subsequent positive patient outcome, client satisfaction and positive practice reputation:

- providing an appointment with a VHCT member that lasts more than ten minutes
- recording nutritional recommendations in the clinical record
- using multiple approaches to client education and communication
- providing written care plans
- providing printed educational material
- reviewing issues covered during the visit, by an appropriately trained member of the team or client relations specialist
- scheduling future appointment before the client leaves the practice
- scheduling follow-up calls, appointments and reminders for ongoing management, to reassess the pet's body weight and condition, and to follow-up on adherence to nutritional recommendations.

Through digital communication and telemedicine, direct client engagement can change the course of a patient's outcome and is something that all members of the VHCT can get involved in. This helps to build the relationship between clients, pets, the VHCT and veterinary practice, increasing the chances of clients seeking advice from the VHCT, rather than from unqualified individuals and inaccurate information sources. It also helps to ensure compliance, which can only be achieved when the nutritional recommendation is well accepted by the client and followed through. Offering virtual weight management consultations can be more convenient for caretakers, avoid potentially stressful car journeys for pets and make nutrition conversations easier. It also enables important information to be captured and enables the communication and reiteration of a nutrition plan and recommendation to all family members. However, a monthly physical examination and NA should be conducted in person until the target weight and BCS is achieved.

Suggestions for future practice

- Regardless of age at the time of surgery, neutering reduces the calorie intake of dogs and cats by 24–33% due to a reduction in basal metabolic rate and/or increased food intake (Eirmann, 2016). It is therefore crucial to discuss diet and feeding management with caretakers at the time of their pet's neutering. Post-op neuter checks led by VNs have the following benefits.
  - An appointment with a VN may be less time constrained than one run by a veterinarian. This increases the opportunity for clients to ask questions and discuss concerns (Wiggins, 2016). Caretakers may also be more prepared to disclose information to VNs (Yeates, 2014),

therefore increasing the chances of obtaining a detailed and more accurate nutritional history.

- o Veterinarians are consulted if required but they can otherwise focus on the tasks and responsibilities that cannot be delegated.
- o The health risks of weight gain can be discussed, together with an explanation about how to assess BCS.
- o Caretakers can be educated about appropriate feeding practices so that neutering doesn't result in an undesirable increase in their pet's food intake and subsequent obesity. If indicated, a weight loss plan can be discussed.
- o Clients are invited to return their pet to the practice for a regular review and measurement of body weight and condition, as part of an NA, thus facilitating the prompt identification of any issues and nutritional risk factors.

- Obesity is commonly observed in ageing animals due to a reduction in metabolism so it is also important to engage with caretakers of pets progressing from mature adult to senior life stage and encourage them to book an appointment at a VN-led senior pet clinic. This could be chargeable but the value and long term benefits should be communicated and an introductory offer could be made to encourage attendance.
- Encourage representatives from each role in the practice team to collaborate and design a nutritional recommendation handout for completion by any member of the practice team in accordance with the veterinarian's or VN's nutritional recommendation. This could contain generic information regarding obesity and weight management as well as tailored information, helping to make the provision of information easier and quicker.
- Establish an online support group for clients with overweight and obese pets via the practice's social media pages and website. Caretakers of pets who have successfully lost weight could be invited to act as mentors.

Scenario 5: A puppy with metabolic bone disease

Practice type: Small animal (referral)

The scenario

Apollo, a 5.5-month-old German Shepherd puppy, is referred for a second opinion due to the caretaker's concerns that his legs look abnormal, and he isn't moving properly. Just 14 weeks previously, Apollo visited a first opinion practice for his second vaccination. At this point, a veterinary professional had enquired about the diet being fed but, once realising it was a large breed puppy diet, demonstrated approval and failed to ask any further questions regarding feeding management.

In the waiting area, the receptionist fusses Apollo and enquires about his general health and wellbeing, including diet. As an advocate of home-made, raw-based feeding, the receptionist listens to the client's rationale for their diet choice and voices concerns about 'heavily-processed' commercial pet food.

On physical examination by the veterinarian, Apollo has angular limb deformity with metaphyseal swelling and a stiff gait. His limbs are bowed when non-weight bearing and he also struggles to rise. He weighs 20.7 kg, with a BCS of 5/9 and mild muscle wastage (WSAVA, 2023). The caretaker has not been monitoring Apollo's growth and there is no record of a formal growth monitoring programme on his clinical records.

The veterinarian takes a medical history and a cursory nutritional history. Nutritional risk factors are identified and discussed with the caretaker. One of the VNs is then asked to obtain a more comprehensive nutritional history from the client before admitting Apollo for biochemical analyses and radiographic examination as part of an extended NA.

The caretakers are well-meaning but new to pet ownership. They have done lots of research online and have also taken advice from Apollo's breeder, all of which recommend a commercial large breed growth diet. The caretakers have young children at home and find that Apollo is getting very distracted when feeding. Realising a puppy's high energy requirement and risk of abnormal bone growth, they decide to offer the diet on a free-feed basis to ensure the intake of sufficient nutrients to optimise growth. Ultimately, they are keen to transfer to a raw meat-based diet and currently offer raw, meaty bones every other day to promote good dental health and to help alleviate boredom when Apollo is left home alone.

Radiography reveals reduced bone density, enlarged epiphyseal line and epiphyseal thickening of the ulna and radius. Decreased serum total calcium and phosphorus concentrations and elevated serum alkaline and creatine kinase are detected via serum biochemical analyses. Based on physical, radio-logical and laboratory examination, evaluation of clinical findings and an extended NA, a diagnosis of nutritional secondary hyperparathyroidism and/or rickets is made. The absence of pathologic fractures and irreversible phy-seal damage suggests a good prognosis for Apollo. Correction of the feeding management is the primary treatment, together with restricted activity to prevent spontaneous fractures. Apollo's daily energy requirement is calcu-lated, together with the correct amount of the puppy's existing commercial large breed growth diet, which the caretakers are instructed to feed only on a meal-restricted and portion-controlled basis. The significant health risks associated with raw feeding are also discussed. An appropriate dietary recom-mendation outlining alterations to Apollo's feeding management is verbally communicated to the caretaker and documented in the patient's clinical record. A handout is also supplied, outlining the risks associated with feeding raw meat-based diets, together with advice on how to feed safely and ensure the diet's nutritional adequacy.

Communication

Effective communication is fundamental to establishing a reliable and trustful relationship between colleagues, and between the VHCT and pet caretakers. The selection of appropriate language, style of communication, information exchange process, decision-making support and empowerment of all members of the VHCT to engage in appropriate conversations can impact many outcomes of veterinary care. However, when communicating with clients, it is important to ensure the delivery of a consistent and accurate message from all members of the VHCT (see 'Professional roles and responsibilities', p. 144).

This scenario highlights the importance of obtaining an accurate nutritional history and how appropriate questioning can reduce the chances of malnutrition and avoid diet-related health issues. At the second vaccine appointment, a veterinary professional enquired, 'What diet are you feeding?' This failed to elicit a full or accurate explanation and so vital information regarding food intake and feeding management was missed, resulting in incorrect assumptions being made and the avoidable occurrence of developmental orthopaedic disease. Encouraging caretakers of newly registered puppies and kittens to routinely complete and submit a nutritional history form prior to a veterinary consultation can help to increase the accuracy of information provision. It also helps to normalise nutritional conversations and facilitates the early identification of potential nutritional risk factors, including the feeding of a nutritionally inadequate and imbalanced diet. On arrival at the practice, appropriate questioning by a suitably qualified or trained member of the VHCT, using a combination of open and closed questions, can be used to obtain a narrative nutritional history (Ward, 2022b). Equal consideration should be given to animal-, diet-, environment-, and human-related factors. Interpretation by a veterinarian or VN, alongside a discussion regarding the pet's breed-specific and life-stage needs can build a stronger relationship and promote the need for preventative care and appropriate diet choices throughout every stage of the pet's life.

Trust and value

Educating about appropriate feeding protocols and diet choice helps to preserve the bond between pets and caretakers. When communicating about pet food decisions and nutritional support, it is essential for the VHCT to understand caretakers' perceptions, attitudes, values and ethical principles to ensure alignment of nutritional and other veterinary recommendations. The caretaker's interest in raw feeding and ultimate desire to transfer their pet to a raw meat-based diet is an important aspiration to explore, particularly given the presence of young children in the household. Growth in the popularity of unconventional diets, and a distrust of commercially produced pet food, increases the risk of feeding a nutritionally inadequate and imbalanced diet, with severe and detrimental consequences to pet health and wellbeing, as well as health and safety concerns for household members. Nutrient deficiencies in dogs and cats fed unbalanced home prepared raw and cooked diets, particularly in kittens and puppies, are widely reported. In contrast to adult animals who are better able to accommodate unbalanced diets and, for whom, clinical signs become evident over a period of years, the effects in growing animals can be seen in just a few weeks. It is thus vital to recognise and manage potential nutritional risk factors. Homemade raw diets can be nutritionally adequate but must be properly balanced through consultation with a DACVIM (Nutrition) Board Certified Veterinary Nutritionist or EBVS European Specialist in Veterinary and Comparative Nutrition.

Clients' pet food philosophies often closely follow their personal food choices (Ward, 2002c) and for this caretaker could include the commitment to only feeding the freshest foods. Understanding the context for clients' pet feeding behaviour, alongside considering and respecting personal values, beliefs, concerns and goals, is essential for achieving consensus and concordance in relation to nutritional, and other veterinary, recommendations. Many perceptions surrounding raw feeding, such as less processing and higher quality, are anecdotal with a limited supporting evidence base. Stressing misguided beliefs helps to reinforce them but not all caretakers will be successfully influenced or persuaded to alter their pet's diet or feeding management. Keeping a detailed record of the NA and recommendation in the patient's clinical record and being proactive in conducting repeated assessments can prompt ongoing discussion and help to demonstrate the VHCT's desire to achieve the best for the pet, their caretaker and family members. It also acknowledges the VHCT's awareness and recognition of the One Health concept and interconnection between people, animals and the environment they share.

Professional roles and responsibilities

It is a responsibility of every member of the veterinary practice team to promote optimal nutrition, provide reliable information and signpost clients to credible further information sources. Effective communication skills and the VHCT's ability to clearly explain the reasons for recommendations drives clients' perceptions of the value and quality of care (Lue *et al.*, 2008). Such findings emphasise the importance of ensuring that each team member provides a positive communication experience with clients and a seamless service.

In this scenario, the receptionist shows great interest in the pet and caretaker, helping to create a positive first impression and the establishment of a personal and emotional connection. Discussing diet and nutrition at every veterinary visit can enhance clients' understanding and attitudes toward veterinary care and highlight the support available from the VHCT in decision-making (Hansen, 2021). However, the influence of cognitive bias in decision-making is great and people hold their own values and beliefs with a high degree of conviction that they are 'right'. Pet caretakers will therefore gravitate towards sources of information most closely aligned to these, even if they are inaccurate and misinformed. As an advocate of homemade, raw-based feeding, the receptionist has personal concerns about commercial pet food, mainly linked to beliefs that it is expensive, yet low quality, and contains dubious ingredients such as animal by-products and waste products. While a willingness to share (nutrition-related) personal experiences can help to enhance VHCT–client communication (Pun, 2020), non-clinical staff should avoid sharing subjective, clinical views with clients which may contradict the recommendation of a vet or VN, or which go against the practice's nutrition protocol and feeding philosophy. It is therefore important to ensure that all practice team members receive appropriate nutritional training, focus on facts and evidence-based practice, avoid imparting their own personal views and biases, and address any client distrust in veterinary advice.

Reflection and evaluation

In this scenario, metabolic bone disease (likely nutritional secondary hyper-parathyroidism and/or rickets) resulted from feeding a nutritionally incomplete and nutrient imbalanced diet. The feeding management is also incorrect, as free feeding can favour the manifestation of other developmental orthopaedic diseases associated with an excessively fast rate of growth. The growth period of large and giant breeds of dog is prolonged, making them susceptible to developmental orthopaedic disease and sensitive to nutrient deficiencies and excesses, altered calcium phosphorus ratio and overfeeding. A diet formulated for large-breed growth, fed on a meal restricted or portion-controlled basis, not ad-libitum, and without any supplementation (especially with minerals), is fundamental to reducing this risk.

It is critical to identify animals at risk of malnutrition through detailed NA and to ensure that diet choice matches the recommended nutrient profile for the species, life stage and lifestyle. Regular NA during growth ensures that dietary adjustments can be made as necessary to encourage gradual growth, managed weight gain and the maintenance of a lean body condition. A formal growth monitoring programme, including the record of body weight and completion of an evidence-based growth chart, such as those provided by Waltham (2022), is recommended monthly during the first six months of life, and then every two to three months until skeletal maturity (German, 2021). This scenario also emphasises the importance of ensuring effective communication of a dietary recommendation and long-term nutritional plan to pet caretakers – and confirming their understanding of the rationale for this.

Encouraging routine and regular pet visits to the veterinary practice during the growth period and beyond facilitates the development of a strong, personal relationship between caretaker, pet and VHCT. It can also help to expand the role of the VHCT beyond the scope of medical provider, enabling the provision of guidance in important areas of proactive care, including diet, exercise, behaviour and the selection of pet products (Hansen, 2021).

Suggestions for future practice

- Produce client friendly materials and resources to help educate on the potential benefits and limitations of feeding a raw and/or homemade diet. Include information on hygiene and the safe handling of pet food, a list of recommended diet brands for clients wanting to feed a commercially produced raw diet, and further information for those wanting to feed a homemade diet. Also make use of existing, freely available resources, such as those produced by WSAVA (2023) and UK Pet Food (2023).
- Design and publish practice policies relating to infectious disease and the hospitalisation of patients fed raw meat-based diets, with a focus on maintaining the health and safety of other patients and staff. This must consider patients that are admitted for elective procedures as well as those admitted as an emergency. It is essential to ensure that such policies are clearly communicated to, and discussed with, clients.

Scenario 6: A cat hospitalised following a road traffic collision

Practice type: Small animal (first opinion)

The scenario

A 12-year male neutered domestic shorthair cat is discovered one evening at the side of the road, unable to walk, presumed to have been hit by a car. He is transported to the veterinary practice by a member of the public and examined out of hours by the duty veterinarian and VN. He has a head tilt and is hyper salivating and rolling to the right. Physical examination reveals nystagmus, blood in the right ear and severe right-sided peripheral vestibular disease secondary to a fractured right bulla and zygomatic arch, with right-sided facial lacerations and a fractured right mandibular canine. He weighs 5.3 kg, has a BCS of 5/9 and a muscle condition score of mild loss. The caretaker is successfully contacted after a scan of the cat's microchip, and he is identified as Milo.

Milo is hospitalised for supportive therapy, including the administration of intravenous fluids and analgesia, monitoring and nursing care. One of the veterinarians, a recent graduate, admits Milo and takes overall responsibility for his initial diagnosis and ongoing treatment. A number of other clinical personnel contribute to his ongoing monitoring, treatment and care provision including qualified VNs, two patient care assistants and a student veterinarian. Over the first 24 hours, Milo is stable and shows some mild improvement of neurological signs, but he continues to roll with any movement, and remains unable to stand. A liquid convalescence diet is offered as it is palatable, energy-dense, easy to consume and supports nutritional restoration and convalescence, yet Milo refuses it. The qualified VNs delegate food provision to the patient care assistants since they spend most time fussing and reassuring patients and have no responsibility for the administration of treatment, thus creating a positive association. This increases the chances of patients feeling relaxed in their company and therefore the likelihood of spontaneous food consumption. The student veterinarian aids the patient care assistants and is tasked with recording Milo's food intake.

Similar signs continue over the next day or so with slow but steady improvement, but still with limited food intake. The patient care assistants use several strategies that have proved successful with previous patients, such as offering the food at room and body temperature, placing the food bowl in a hide box, offering opportunities to eat regularly, and using flat or wide-brimmed bowls, but with limited success. Despite the regular administration of analgesia, pain is investigated as a potential barrier to food intake but dismissed because of frequent pain score results. Other physical and invisible barriers are explored but rejected for various reasons. The veterinarian appears to be unconcerned about Milo's food intake and believes his appetite will return with improvement of neurological function. A VN advises the student veterinarian to contact the caretaker and obtain a nutritional history, including dietary preferences and feeding management and this is replicated, where possible, in the hospital.

The patient care assistants express their increasing concern about Milo's lack of food intake to the qualified VNs and veterinarian. The qualified VNs suggest the implementation of further nutritional support in the form of a feeding tube but the veterinarian is reluctant to place a naso-oesophageal tube due to Milo's facial injuries and feels an oesophagostomy tube is too invasive and unnecessary. Anti-emetics and appetite stimulants are prescribed. Feline food preferences are established at an early age and, when in unfamiliar surroundings, cats can be less tolerant of novel food, such as prescription diets (Taylor *et al.*, 2022). Therefore, the VNs invite the caretakers to visit Milo and to assist in encouraging food intake. Milo consumes a small amount of chicken, and the caretaker suggests continuing with this as it is one of his favourite treats at home.

Continued improvement is seen over the following 72 hours, with Milo spending increasing time in sternal recumbency and demonstrating a willingness to consume small amounts of palatable meats. Yet his limited food intake is thought to be the main contributory factor to weight loss and remains a significant concern. The patient care assistants complain that the issues being raised are being ignored, compromising patient health and welfare, and demonstrating a lack of recognition and appreciation of their views. The student veterinarian also vents frustration and highlights the risk of malnutrition due to inadequate food intake, citing evidence from a recent lecture regarding the relationship between caloric intake and hospital outcome and the impact that positive-energy balance has on patient outcome and discharge time. The VN reports that Milo is failing to meet his daily resting energy requirements and raises concerns about the risk of hepatic lipidosis, but the veterinarian remains reluctant to place a feeding tube and becomes defensive, making further conversations about the patient challenging for team members.

Communication

In veterinary practice, challenging situations, including sources of conflict, often have little to do with the actual practice of veterinary medicine and are more often a result of team members' miscommunication, assumptions and lack of self-control (Charles, 2014). Effective communication is fundamental to the avoidance of miscommunications and misunderstandings. Having an objective language that focuses on factual information, rather than personal opinion and subjective views, helps to build strong channels of communication and avoids creating feelings of criticism or blame.

In this scenario, a record of the patient's nutritional support and food intake was made in his clinical record, yet the team failed to design a nutritional plan and there was no routine daily evaluation to support the continuum of care and provision of enteral nutritional support. The patient was hand-fed small amounts of chicken and other palatable meat, potentially leading to an incorrect assumption that his nutrition was being adequately addressed. However, hand feeding is often time-consuming, rarely sufficient to meet a patient's energy or nutrient requirements, and often delays the implementation of nutritional support (Gajanayake, 2014). The lack of agreement regarding the patient's nutritional care resulted in interprofessional conflict and tension between team members. One member of the team had differing views to the remainder of the team, ultimately resulting in team division, communication breakdown, potential isolation of that team member and a difficult future working relationship.

When faced with a situation involving opposing views, not all team members will speak up. Yet concealing frustrations can interfere with performance and attitude, ultimately making it difficult to be an invested team member and contribute to the overarching shared goal of the VHCT and practice mission (Dobbs, 2013). As outlined by Hunter and Shaw (2015), the use of differing opinions can provide an opportunity to collaborate, and problem-solve by:

- recognising the value of different views and mind-sets
- asking colleagues how they would handle the situation, so their opinion is respected and acknowledged
- focusing on working towards the common goal and achieving the best for the patient (and caretaker)

- using inclusive language to communicate effectively, such as 'let's', 'we', 'our' and 'together'
- defining a practice culture which supports its team members in speaking out and challenging the current situation in an appropriate manner, providing constructive suggestions for improvement
- using positive and receptive non-verbal communication, which can further encourage team members to share and clarify their perspectives, beliefs and concerns.

Trust and value

In veterinary practice, pet caretakers and members of the VHCT will have different perspectives, values, beliefs and goals which can escalate into conflict and emotional turmoil. Conflict is a part of life that is hard to avoid and is therefore considered an inevitable part of any workplace (Kerrigan, 2019). This scenario presents a shared ethical position with the aim of all team members to provide the patient with the highest quality of care and meet the client's needs, however interprofessional conflict arises as a result of contrasting viewpoints and beliefs.

- **Patient welfare and prevention of suffering**. 'Not eating' is universally considered a poor quality of life and while this clinical presentation is common, it has significant consequences for patients, client retention and the practice's health (Marks, 2022). As outlined in the 2006 Animal Welfare Act (Gov.UK, 2022), anyone with responsibility for an animal has a duty of care to ensure that the animal's needs are met and that it doesn't suffer unnecessarily. In most, if not all, jurisdictions, a failure to provide adequate nutrition equates to unnecessary suffering and, while the VHCT did not withhold food from the patient, it is immoral to permit starvation. A reduced or absent appetite in hospitalised patients results in 'stressed starvation'. This hypermetabolic state is associated with increased energy expenditure and proteolysis, and accelerated loss of lean body mass (Taylor *et al.*, 2022). Deleterious effects of starvation, including increased mortality rates, become more pronounced after three days of appetite decline (Gagne and Wakshlag, 2015), therefore, for many patients, nutritional support should be instigated as soon as possible.
- **Low appreciation and lack of mutual respect and trust**. The extent to which staff feel valued directly affects the degree to which clients feel valued, directly impacting business success (Flamholtz, 2001). Getting to know and empowering colleagues, identifying their strengths and knowledge, demonstrating a willingness to learn and understand other roles, and being open to questions and constructive feedback can help to develop and build effective working relationships and mutual trust and appreciation (Vande Linde, 2017).

This scenario also highlights the importance of developing trust between patients and the VHCT. Building trust and the bond between patients and members of the VHCT can help to create positive associations for patients and may improve the chances of them spontaneously eating (Collins, 2016).

Professional roles and responsibilities

Many veterinary practices have a number of individuals performing a variety of patient- and client-oriented tasks. With increasing professional diversity, the functionality of veterinary professionals, including veterinarians and VNs, and support staff, must be predicated on positive relationships. Embracing all members of the VHCT, including diverse individual and professional perspectives, at all stages of patient care is fundamental to the integration of NA and the optimisation of nutritional care.

The team environment in this scenario turned increasingly negative with resulting dissatisfaction, stress and frustration felt by team members. Knowing, connecting and communicating with other members in the team in an open and non-judgemental way is essential to optimising long-term care of the patient. All roles in the VHCT have responsibility as an advocate for the patient and have an overarching shared goal to provide the best patient and client care. By working toward this common goal, the team can develop a better understanding of the key role they each play and how their roles are interdependent (Hunter and Shaw, 2015).

Veterinarian

Conversations about deeply-held beliefs are often emotional and those involved can easily become defensive (Bateman, 2016). Ultimately, the veterinarian is striving for the best patient outcome but colleagues' attribution of blame and questioning of clinical decision-making ability may result in feelings of being undermined and distrusted. There are a number of potential reasons behind the veterinarian's reluctance to place a feeding tube including the patient's condition, risk of complications, requirement for a general anaesthetic and cost. As a recent graduate, concerns over confidence, knowledge, skills and expertise required to complete the procedure could also be a realistic concern. Veterinarians in the early postgraduate period cite inadequate mentorship and support as the second most important determinant for leaving a place of employment (Jelinski *et al.*, 2009), a factor that is also associated with increased workplace stress, particularly in female employees (Heath, 1997).

VNs

Providing optimal nutrition to hospitalised patients is often considered a duty of care for VNs and yet, despite their awareness of the importance of nutrition and the effects of malnutrition on a patient, this doesn't guarantee that inpatients will receive appropriate nutritional support (Cox, 2020). Veterinarians and VNs have shared responsibilities and must coordinate the care of patients and delivery of veterinary services, but with an understanding and recognition of the scope and limitations of their role. In this scenario, the VN identifies that the patient is at risk of undernutrition and is concerned about the negative consequences but isn't comfortable questioning the veterinarian's decision-making in relation to a procedure that VNs must be knowledgeable about, but are insufficiently qualified to perform.

Patient care assistants and student veterinarian

Both the patient care assistants and the student veterinarian are confident to speak up and motivated to do so out of concern for the patient and perceived risk of malnutrition. The student veterinarian believes that sound scientific evidence is paramount and is enthusiastic about applying theory to practice, yet maybe fails to consider the many other factors that influence clinical decision-making. Student veterinarians and student VNs are trained to challenge information, concepts and ideas. Their views can therefore be central to the examination and evaluation of traditional methods, practice and policies and to changing behaviour and practice. However, it is essential that concerns and differences in opinion are raised in a professional and respectful manner and one which promotes a constructive outcome.

Reflection and evaluation

Nutritional care is one of the most fundamental aspects of veterinary healthcare and plays a crucial role in improving patient outcomes, increasing chances of survival and reducing discharge time. While there is a growing recognition of the importance of nutrition in veterinary medicine, the adequacy of nutritional care in veterinary practice continues to be questioned (Bergler *et al.*, 2016; Santarossa *et al.*, 2018; Bruckner and Handl, 2020; Alvarez *et al.*, 2022) and the incidence of undernutrition in veterinary patients is often underestimated (Remillard *et al.*, 2001; Brunetto *et al.*, 2010; Molina *et al.*, 2018).

In this scenario, the presence of a number of risk factors put Milo at an increased risk of malnutrition (Perea, 2012), including:

- an insufficient food intake to meet at least 80% of the daily resting energy requirement
- weight loss
- a muscle condition score of mild loss
- an expected course of illness lasting several days.

This causes concern for the VNs and support staff involved in his care, with subsequent team conflict regarding ongoing nutritional support. Confronting interprofessional and interpersonal conflict in a team can be challenging and upsetting, but unresolved conflict can prove damaging to the veterinary team and practice, and its patients and clients. Addressing conflict in an appropriate and professional manner will ultimately result in improved working relationships, a more productive environment and empowerment of the team (Kerrigan, 2019).

Suggestions for future practice

This situation occurred in a small first opinion veterinary practice that rarely accommodates long-stay patients. Consequently, a number of fundamental care components were overlooked, including the following.

- The generation of a nutrition plan with input from veterinarians, VNs, patient care assistants, students and other relevant members of the VHCT. This should be subject to continuous assessment, planning, implementation and evaluation. While implicit care planning often comes naturally, it is important to explicitly plan patient care and create a detailed nutrition plan, in addition to a nursing care plan.
- The provision of daily ward rounds with representation across different roles to discuss the condition and ongoing care and treatment requirements of hospitalised patients. Open discussions involving all clinical team members can help to ensure that patient and client needs are met, reduce the incidence of preventable events and proactively address any reported issues.

Further suggestions for future practice include the following.

- Utilisation of an assessment tool to identify patients' need for nutritional support.
- Design and implementation of a practice policy on the nutritional support of hospitalised patients which is subject to an annual review. This must be clearly communicated and consistently applied to all team members who are then accountable for its implementation and use.
- Completion of a clinical audit on the number of patients for whom nutritional support is delayed. The use of nutrition plans can prove a valuable tool for retrospective clinical audits to support clinical governance.
- Implementation of weekly team meetings to ensure that all members have an opportunity to raise, discuss and address any perceived challenges or issues, for example, in relation to the completion of their role or a practice policy.
- Provision of processes for team members to constructively deal with issues and engage in conflict resolution.
- Creation of training exercises, such as 'Talking Walls' (Kinnison *et al.*, 2012), to help raise awareness and appreciation of the roles and contribution of team members.
- Provision of training to enhance communication skills and to help minimise and resolve conflict.

In summary

As illustrated in this chapter and throughout this publication, a proactive team-based approach is fundamental to the optimisation of patient care and treatment and the provision of nutritional advice, care and support in veterinary practice. Irregularity in the completion of a full NA is likely to result in undetected nutritional risk factors, with significant consequences for patient care and a reactive, instead of a proactive, attitude towards nutrition. A consistent and detailed approach, involving all members of the VHCT, is fundamental to effective NA and support, and the provision of dietary recommendations and protocols. By working together and utilising the many freely available tools to make nutritional conservation and assessment easier and faster, many of the acknowledged challenges in implementation can be overcome.

References

AAHA (American Animal Hospital Association) (2009) *Compliance: Taking Quality Care to the Next Level: A Report of the 2009 AAHA Compliance Follow-up Study*. AAHA Press, Lakewood, Colorado.

Alvarez, E.E., Schultz, K.K., Floerchinger, A.M. and Hull, J.L. (2022) Small animal general practitioners discuss nutrition infrequently despite assertion of indication, citing barriers. *Journal of the American Veterinary Medical Association,* 260(13), 1704–1710.

Bateman, S. (2016) Addressing diverse beliefs with courageous conversations. Available at: https://www.cliniciansbrief.com/article/addressing-diverse-beliefs-courageous-conversations (accessed 15 December 2022).

Bergler, R., Wechsung, S., Kienzle, E., Hoff, T. and Dobenecker, B. (2016) Nutrition consultation in small animal practice – a field for specialized veterinarians. *Tierarztl Prax Ausg K Kleintiere Heimtiere,* 44, 5–14.

Boatright, K. (2020) The cost of caring too much? *Today's Veterinary Practice,* 10(1), 86–88.

Bruckner, I. and Handl, S. (2020) Survey on the role of nutrition in first-opinion practices in Austria and Germany: An evaluation of knowledge, preferences and need for further education. *Journal of Animal Physiology and Animal Nutrition,* 105 (Suppl. 2), 89–94.

Brunetto, M.A., Gomes, M.O.S., Andre, M. R., Teshima, E., Gonçalves, K.N. *et al.* (2010) Effects of nutritional support on hospital outcome in dogs and cats. *Journal of Veterinary Emergency and Critical Care,* 20, 224–231.

Charles, E. (2014) What is emotional intelligence & why does it matter in veterinary medicine? Available at: https://www.cliniciansbrief.com/article/what-emotional-intelligence-why-does-it-matter-veterinary-medicine (accessed 14 December 2022).

Collins, S. (2016) The importance of nutrition in the post-operative recovery of cats and dogs. *Veterinary Nursing Journal,* 31(8), 233–236.

Cox, S. (2020) A holistic approach to creating a nutrition plan for hospitalised inpatients. *The Veterinary Nurse,* 11(3), 126–131.

Davies, M. (2022) Obesity: long-term strategies for weight issues in cats and dogs. *Vet Times*, 52(35), 6–8.

Dobbs, K. (2013) Practice policy: how to handle a difference of opinion. Available at: https://www.cliniciansbrief.com/article/practice-policy-how-handle-difference-opinion (accessed 14 December 2022).

Eirmann, L. (2016) Nutritional assessment. *Veterinary Clinics of North America: Small Animal Practice,* 46(5), 855–867.

Flamholtz, E. (2001) Corporate culture and the bottom line. *European Management Journal*, 19(3), 268–275.

Freeman, L., Becvarova, I., Cave, N., MacKay, C., Nguyen, P. *et al.* (2011) WSAVA nutritional assessment guidelines. *Journal of Small Animal Practice*, 52(7), 385–396.

Gagne, J.W. and Wakshlag, J.J. (2015) Pathophysiology and clinical approach to malnutrition in dogs and cats. In: Chan, D.L. (ed.) *Nutritional Management of Hospitalised Small Animals*. Wiley Blackwell, Chichester, UK, pp. 117–127.

Gajanayake, I. (2014) Management of the anorexic cat. *In Practice*, 36, 163–171.

German, A. (2021). Association between canine body condition and lifespan. *Veterinary Times*, 51(7), 7–8.

Gov.UK (2022) Animal welfare. Available at: https://www.gov.uk/guidance/animal-welfare (accessed 20 December 2022)

Hansen, C. (2021) Stronger client relationships are key to better patient care. *dvm360*, 55(5), 25–26.

Heath, T. (1997) Experiences and attitudes of recent veterinary graduates: A national survey. *Australian Veterinary Practitioner*, 27, 45–50.

Hodgkiss, B.A., Lo, A.W.F., Loney, C.L., Wickers, A.S.J. and Yam, P.S. (2020) What's weighing on your mind? A novel approach to canine weight management. Presented at the 4th annual INSPIRE Research Forum, January 22 2020, Glasgow, UK.

Hunter, L. and Shaw, J. (2015) Tips for team communication. Available at: https://www.cliniciansbrief.com/article/tips-team-communication (accessed 16 November 2022).

Janke, N., Coe, J.B., Bernardo, T.M., Dewey, C.E. and Stone, E.A. (2021) Pet owners' and veterinarians' perceptions of information exchange and clinical decision-making in companion animal practice. *PLoS ONE,* 16(2): e0245632.

Janke, N., Shaw, J.R., and Coe, J.B. (2022) Veterinary technicians contribute to shared decision-making during companion animal veterinary appointments. *Journal of the American Veterinary Medical Association*, 260(15), 1993–2000.

Jelinski, M.D., Campbell, J.R., MacGregor and M.W., Watts, J.M. (2009) Factors associated with veterinarians' career path choices in the early postgraduate period. *Canadian Veterinary Journal*, 50(9), 943–948.

Johnson, J. (2022) The importance of the human–animal bond for the veterinary profession. Available at: https://habri.org/hab-lectures?view-session=the-importance-of-the-human-animal-bond-for-the-veterinary-profession (accessed 19 June 2022).

Kerrigan, L. (2019) Strategies for managing conflict within a team. *The Veterinary Nurse*, 10(6), 292–295.

Kinnison, T., Lumbis, R.H., Orpet, H., Welsh, P., Gregory, S.P. and Baillie, S. (2012).How to run Talking Walls: An interprofessional education resource. *The Veterinary Nurse*, 3, 4–11.

Kipperman, B.S. and German, A.J. (2018) The responsibility of veterinarians to address companion animal obesity. *Animals (Basel)*, 8(9), 143.

Lavoie, J.P. (2020) *Blackwell's Five-Minute Veterinary Consult: Equine*, 3rd edn. Wiley Blackwell, New Jersey, USA.

Linder, D. (2021) Compliance strategies for the obese patient. *Today's Veterinary Practice*, 11(3), 36–39.

Lue, T.W., Pantenburg, D.P. and Crawford, P.M. (2008) Impact of the owner–pet and client–veterinarian bond on the care that pets receive. *Journal of the American Veterinary Medical Association*, 232, 531–540.

Marks, N. (2022) Take a bite out of inappetence. *Today's Veterinary Business*, 6(1), 66–67.

Mattson, K. (2021) Nutritional conversations, front and center. Available at: https://www.avma.org/javma-news/2021-07-01/nutritional-conversations-front-and-center (accessed 10 November 2022).

Miller, C. (2022) Small mammal herbivores part 3: taking a dietary history and providing nutritional support. *The Veterinary Nurse*, 13(9), 417–425.

Molina, J., Hervera, M., Manzanilla, E.G., Torrente, C. and Villaverde, C. (2018) Evaluation of the prevalence and risk factors for undernutrition in hospitalized dogs. *Frontiers in Veterinary Science*, 5, 205.

Perea, S.C. (2012) Parenteral nutrition. In: Fascetti, A.J. and Delaney, S.J. (eds) *Applied Veterinary Clinical Nutrition*. Wiley Blackwell, Chichester, UK, pp. 353–373.

PFMA (2015) Guinea pig size-o-meter. Available at: https://pfma.carbonit.co.uk/guinea-pig-size-o-meter (accessed 04 December 2022).

Pirie, R.S. and McGorum, B.C. (2018) Equine grass sickness: an update. *UK-Vet Equine*, 2(1), 6–10.

Porsani, M.Y.H., Teixeira, F.A., Amaral, A.R., Pedrinelli, V., Vasques, V. *et al.* (2020) Factors associated with failure of dog's weight loss programmes. *Veterinary Medicine and Science*, 6(3), 299–305.

Pun, J.K.H. (2020) An integrated review of the role of communication in veterinary clinical practice. *BMC Veterinary Research*, 16(394), 1–14.

Quesenberry, K.E. and Carpenter, J. (2012) *Ferrets, Rabbits, and Rodents: Clinical Medicine and Surgery*, 3rd edn. Elsevier Saunders, St. Louis, Missouri, pp. 279–284.

RCVS (2022) Code of professional conduct for veterinary nurses. Available at: https://www.rcvs.org.uk/setting-standards/advice-and-guidance/code-of-professional-conduct-for-veterinary-nurses/ (accessed 19 November 2022).

Remillard, R.L., Darden, D.E., Michel, K.E., Marks, S.L., Buffington, C.A. *et al.* (2001) An investigation of the relationship between caloric intake and outcome in hospitalised dogs. *Veterinary Therapeutics*, 2, 301–310.

Rowe, E.C., Browne, W.J., Casey, R.A., Gruffydd-Jones, T.J. and Murray, J.K. (2017) Early-life risk factors identified for owner-reported feline overweight and obesity at around two years of age. *Preventive Veterinary Medicine*, 143, 39–48.

Santarossa, H.A., Parr, J.M. and Verbrugghe, A. (2018) Assessment of canine and feline body composition by veterinary healthcare teams in Ontario, Canada. *Canadian Veterinary Journal*, 59, 1280–1286.

Taylor, S., Chan D.L., Villaverde, C., Ryan, L., Person, F. *et al.* (2022) 2022 ISFM consensus guidelines on management of the inappetent hospitalised cat. *Journal of Feline Medicine and Surgery*, 24(7), 614–640.

Troyer, H. and Goodman Lee, J. (2013) Clinical suite: Obesity in dogs & cats. Available at: https://www.cliniciansbrief.com/article/clinical-suite-obesity-dogs-cats (accessed 11 December 2022).

UK Pet Food (2023) Resource library. Available at: https://www.ukpetfood.org/information-centre/all-uk-pet-food-resources.html (accessed 1 January 2023).

Vande Linde, M.A. (2017) Focus on teamwork to kick the cliques. Available at: https://www.cliniciansbrief.com/article/focus-teamwork-kick-cliques (accessed 18 December 2022).

Wainwright, J., Millar, K.M. and White, G.A. (2022) Owners' views of canine nutrition, weight status and wellbeing and their implications for the veterinary consultation. *Journal of Small Animal Practice*, 63, 381–388.

Waltham (2022) WALTHAM™ Puppy Growth Charts. Available at: https://www.waltham.com/resources/puppy-growth-charts (accessed 10 April 2023).

Ward, E. (2022a) Consistency creates credibility. *Today's Veterinary Business*, 6(2), 14–17.

Ward, E. (2022b) How to expand the pet food conversation. *Today's Veterinary Business*, 6(3), 12–15.

Ward, E. (2022c) How to not talk like a salesperson. *Today's Veterinary Business*, 6(4), 10–13.

Wiggins, H. (2016) How to run a successful nurse clinic. *The Veterinary Nurse*, 7(5), 286–290.

WSAVA (2023) Global nutrition toolkit. Available at: https://wsava.org/Global-Guidelines/Global-Nutrition-Guidelines/ (accessed 1 January 2023).

Yeates, J. (2014) The role of the veterinary nurse in animal welfare. *Veterinary Nursing Journal*, 29(7), 250–251.

Interprofessional learning and education

10

Tierney Kinnison

Abstract

Interprofessional education (IPE) relates to two or more professions learning together to improve collaboration and care. IPE can relate to both undergraduate and postgraduate education (continuing professional development or CDP), as well as incorporating both formal and informal elements, such as the hidden curriculum. IPE is relatively rare in the veterinary field, which fails to portray to our students and graduates the importance of this aspect of their future work. Initiatives from human medicine and veterinary medicine are provided as examples in order to encourage the development of IPE which focuses on veterinary nutrition, with an underlying concept of teamwork. While individuals with a special interest in nutrition may choose nutrition-related CPD, many professionals whose specialist interests lie elsewhere may not, thus encouragement and promotion to partake in interprofessional nutrition CPD may be important.

Naturally, training is required for members of the veterinary healthcare team (VHCT) to have the required nutritional knowledge and interprofessional teamwork skills to form teams which can provide optimum nutritional care to patients and caretakers. As explored in Chapter 8, it is important for the nutrition-related training needs of the VHCT to be identified and for all team members to undergo training on the key points of the practice's philosophy on nutrition. This is in addition to ensuring that the clinical team members complete appropriate continuing professional development (CPD) and continuing education (CE) regarding nutrition, alongside other aspects of practice. The time required for this training, therefore, needs to be understood and facilitated by the practice's management team.

However, as educators of members of professions providing a public service, we can do more at an earlier stage to ensure a smooth transition to interprofessional nutritional practice upon graduation. Interprofessional education (IPE) has been defined as occurring 'when students from two or more professions learn about, from and with each other to enable effective collaboration and improve health outcomes' (WHO, 2010). IPE is still relatively rare in the veterinary field, but has been developed and researched in the fields of aviation and human healthcare which, as identified in Chapter 1 of this book, have been the forerunners with regard to interprofessional working and learning.

IPE is very varied, with the types of teaching methods (including didactic or interactive) varying between institutions, and the different disciplines conducting, and being involved in, the initiatives (Herath *et al.*, 2017). Questions for the existing literature in the pioneer disciplines, therefore, are 'Does IPE work?' and 'What aspects of IPE work?'. There have been several systematic reviews in recent years which have sought to explore these questions, and to help institutions develop effective IPE initiatives. A few examples are included in Table 10.1.

Although reporting bias may have led to an over-representation of studies with positive results of IPE, in comparison to no significant differences, or negative impacts of IPE interventions, the systematic reviews below should encourage veterinary educators to develop and implement IPE in the teaching of their undergraduate students. Further research is still required to evaluate the impact of undergraduate IPE on future changes in behaviour and impacts on

Table 10.1. Recent systematic reviews aiming to identify the benefits of IPE, presented chronologically.

Authors	Article title	Main findings
Reeves *et al.*, 2016	A BEME systematic review of the effects of interprofessional education: BEME Guide No. 39	**46 articles included** Positive outcomes were reported more often than negative or neutral outcomes, including learners responding well to IPE, improvement in attitudes and perceptions of each other, and reported increases in knowledge and skills.
Guraya and Barr, 2018	The effectiveness of interprofessional education in healthcare: A systematic review and meta-analysis	**12 articles included** Meta-analysis shows a positive impact and effectiveness (in terms of students' knowledge, skills and attitudes) due to IPE interventions in various disciplines
Kangas *et al.*, 2018	An integrative systematic review of interprofessional education on diabetes	**14 articles included** Achieved outcomes were individual gain and external benefits (patients). Experiences of IPE incorporated both challenges and strengths.
Dyess *et al.*, 2019	Impact of interprofessional education on students of the health professions: A systematic review	**7 articles included** All articles reported positive impact on students, including improving teamwork, communication and shared problem-solving.

practice (Reeves *et al.*, 2016). However, these are extremely difficult areas to research due in part to challenges with attributing change in practice to specific IPE initiatives. In addition, it is important to include context in considerations of the optimum IPE, and therefore veterinary-specific research is important.

The authors of this book have been involved in several articles describing the development of veterinary IPE and researching its impact on the students involved. In the work by Kinnison and colleagues described throughout this book (Kinnison *et al.*, 2015a, 2015b, 2015c, 2016) the authors sought to explore interprofessional working in practice to guide future IPE initiatives. Lessons learnt included the importance of opportunities to develop trust and respect between the professions, to further the understanding of each other's roles prior to graduation and to highlight the importance of communication, including speaking up. Additional articles have evaluated specific interventions, such as those asking students to think of and discuss roles and responsibilities, and to practise teamwork, such as cardiopulmonary-cerebral resuscitation (Kinnison *et al.*, 2011). These have also reported on preliminary testing of new tools to evaluate IPE in the veterinary field (Kinnison *et al.*, 2021).

In 2021, the authors of this book and their colleagues wrote a teaching tip regarding developing IPE for veterinarians and veterinary nurses (VNs) (Lumbis *et al.*, 2021). In this article, we outline the importance of utilising educational theories when developing new IPE initiatives, as well as the requirement for both time and financial support for and from faculty. The article also describes how, in the Royal Veterinary College (RVC), we have developed a staff and student team who work to deliver IPE both as part of and in addition to the curricula of the college. The student-led team has been invaluable in raising awareness of IPE in the student body, in gaining external funding and speakers for events, and for continuing to drive forwards the RVC's ability to create the best provision and opportunities for their diverse student body, including veterinary students, veterinary nursing students and bioscience students. One teaching initiative which is described in the teaching tip relates to interprofessional dentistry to address the limited, and siloed, teaching of dentistry to veterinarians and VNs in the UK. Voluntary workshops allow students to develop skills in using dental equipment, understand the charting procedure using models, and recognise the interprofessional roles within dentistry. Other veterinary research has also exposed students' desire for IPE, including a study from Germany which identified that 76% of veterinary students, veterinary assistant trainees and animal keeper trainees would like to partake in interprofessional communication training, and thought that it would aid cooperation with future colleagues (91%), though interestingly only half thought it would help them to respect their future colleagues (53%) (Rauch *et al.*, 2021). Educators should therefore aim to research the desire, practicalities and pedagogical requirements of teaching communication with caretakers and with colleagues in an interprofessional way, in addition to the possibility of teaching other important and mutually relevant topics.

As this book has demonstrated nutrition is an ideal topic for the consideration of interprofessional teamworking. With this in mind, in 2018, a student-led team at the RVC delivered a very successful event called 'The Interprofessional Club Weight Clinic Evening', involving guest speaker lecturers and small-group clinical discussions, sponsored by Hill's Pet Nutrition. However, aside from this one-off event IPE regarding nutrition in the veterinary field appears somewhat non-existent.

In human healthcare, it is possible to identify several articles describing IPE initiatives which focus on, or include, nutritional elements. This highlights how nutrition is a vital part of many interactions with caretakers/patients, including for example complex and long-term healthcare. The fundamental difference between the examples from healthcare and those from veterinary medicine is that healthcare studies include specific nutrition and dietetics students, who will naturally have a greater understanding of the nutritional components of the IPE course than their other professional colleagues. The Academy of Nutrition and Dietetics has made a statement that registered dietitian nutritionists should play a significant role in the education of other professions in undergraduate education and practice (Hark and Deen, 2017), while it is also important to note that this is a two-way interaction, and IPE also leads to better knowledge of dietetics students regarding other professions which can impact future learning including placements (Earland *et al.*, 2011). A selection of IPE examples from healthcare are presented in Table 10.2. It may be possible for educators to adapt and develop aspects of these examples for a veterinary education context.

In addition to the formal IPE delivered as part of curricula and offered as extracurricular activities, it is important to remember the impact of informal learning in terms of role models and hidden curricula. The 'hidden curriculum' relates to attitudes and behaviours learned by students that are unintended, and is in contrast to the formal, taught, curriculum; it has been explored within medical education by Hafferty and Castellani (2019). It can relate to what is notably missing, and in all courses involving veterinary or veterinary nursing education, the majority of teaching will be uni-professional, i.e. students in each discipline working in isolation from each other, and from other groups and professions such as farriers, equine dentists and animal behaviourists. This in itself sends our students the message that they are separate from each other, that they should learn to work by themselves, and should develop teamworking skills within their profession only. By increasing the frequency, visibility and importance of IPE (including assessing interprofessional competences), we will start to send the right messages regarding the importance of working as an interprofessional team.

The hidden curriculum and role models are relevant to what happens in all forms of learning, from didactic lectures to practicals and placements. In their exploration of team communications in the operating room, Lingard *et al.* (2002) describe 'higher-tension events', with the most frequent of these occurring between surgical and nursing staff. They subsequently explain how surgical trainees will either withdraw from a higher-tension event, for example by walking away from a discussion, or instead mimic a senior member of staff,

Table 10.2. Example IPE initiatives regarding nutrition from human medicine, presented chronologically.

Authors	Article title	Teaching initiative	Further information
Pullon *et al.,* 2013	Interprofessional education for physiotherapy, medical and dietetics students: a pilot programme	Time: a course (specific time frame unknown) Students: 21 (7 each of dietetic, physiotherapy and medical students) Details: Learning outcomes included respectful, open communication, patient-centred collaboration, mutually satisfactory negotiation and renegotiation, and shared decision-making. Activities included meet and greet, interactive session, online discussion, home visit, group presentation including management plan	Survey and focus groups used to evaluate learning and change in attitudes. Results indicate increase in positive interprofessional attitudes and confidence.
O'Shea *et al.,* 2019	Using simulation-based learning to provide interprofessional education in diabetes to nutrition and dietetics and exercise physiology students through telehealth	Time: 90 min. plus pre-reading Students: 10 nutrition and dietetics students and 13 exercise physiology students participated Details: Online pre-reading followed by orientation, briefing, simulation, debriefing. Students work in pairs and observe each other's interactions with a patient	Questionnaire scales used to evaluate the initiative. Suggest positive results, especially regarding learning from and about each other.
Khalafalla *et al.,* 2020	Enhancing nutrition and lifestyle education for healthcare professional students through an interprofessional, team-based training program	Time: 4 x 2 hr session Students: 12 PharmD students and 3 dietetic students Details: topics included – obesity, healthy nutrition and lifestyle, coaching and motivational interviewing skills, cultural competency. Included mock interviews with feedback	Basic evaluation using quantitative and qualitative data suggested students had a positive reaction to the training and increased knowledge.
Svensberg *et al.,* 2021	Interprofessional education on complex patients in nursing homes: a focus group study	Time: a course (specific time frame unknown) Students: advanced geriatric nursing, clinical nutrition, dentistry, medicine and pharmacy Details: working in practice-based interprofessional teams in nursing homes	Focus groups conducted to analyse experiences. Results included complex patients creating learning opportunities for students within varied collaborations.

including attitudes, tone of voice and particular wording in demands of other members of the team.

It is important, therefore, if you are working in a veterinary practice which takes student veterinarians and/or student VNs, that you are aware of your own actions, the actions of your team, and the culture of your practice, in promoting the core values of trust, respect and utilisation of each other's skills and knowledge. Further to this, if you take both veterinary and veterinary nursing students, it is beneficial to provide explicit ways for them to work together which may combat the natural tendency for them to feel in competition with each other for the chance to perform desirable tasks, and empower them to be more effective in a VHCT following graduation.

This chapter began with a brief commentary on the importance of CPD and CE regarding nutrition and interprofessional working in an already existing VHCT, and it is worth reiterating this point. CPD focused on nutrition is available and should be utilised, while new and existing CPD should also seek to be inclusive to both clinical professions and to specifically include learning outcomes related to interprofessional working in nutrition cases. Research has suggested that individuals from specific veterinary areas consider their specialisation as being underrepresented in undergraduate education (Kinnison and May, 2013). This may lead to such individuals choosing to undertake CPD primarily in their area of interest, and not to address gaps in knowledge and enhance a holistic approach to care. This may be supported by research from New Zealand suggesting veterinarians most commonly chose CPD based on interest in the topic (Gates *et al.*, 2021). Promotion of nutrition CPD in a VHCT may therefore be required to ensure the team keeps up to date with their knowledge. It is possible that ongoing needs assessment analyses should be conducted with veterinary professionals to explore optimum CPD for VHCTs, as has previously been carried out in dieticians in human medicine (Klevans and Parrett, 1990).

In summary

IPE is a topic which is growing in interest and research in the human and veterinary healthcare fields. Its aims, at both an undergraduate and postgraduate level, to bring together members of different professions to learn together to create better functioning teams, align perfectly with the interprofessional requirements of nutritional care for veterinary patients and their caretakers. Efforts to specifically design nutritional education opportunities which incorporate aspects of IPE, such as roles and responsibilities, trust and respect, and communication are encouraged. Examples provided in this chapter from medicine and veterinary IPE in other topics may be used to guide such initiatives.

References

Dyess, A.L., Brown, J.S., Brown, N.D., Flautt, K.M. and Barnes, L.J. (2019) Impact of interprofessional education on students of the health professions: A systematic review. *Journal of Educational Evaluation for Health Professions*, 16, 1–6.

Earland, J., Gilchrist, M., McFarland, L. and Harrison, K. (2011) Dietetics students' perceptions and experiences of interprofessional education. *Journal of Human Nutrition and Dietetics*, 24(2), 135–143.

Gates, M.C., McLachlan, I., Butler, S. and Weston, J.F. (2021) Practices, preferences, and opinions of New Zealand veterinarians towards continuing professional development. *New Zealand Veterinary Journal*, 69(1), 27–37.

Guraya, S.Y. and Barr, H. (2018) The effectiveness of interprofessional education in healthcare: A systematic review and meta-analysis. *Kaohsiung Journal of Medical Sciences*, 34(3), 160–165.

Hafferty, F. and Castellani, B. (2019) The hidden curriculum: A theory of medical education. In: Brosnan, C. and Turner, B.S. (eds) *Handbook of the Sociology of Medical Education*. Routledge, Oxford, UK, pp. 15–35.

Hark, L.A. and Deen, D. (2017) Position of the Academy of Nutrition and Dietetics: Interprofessional education in nutrition as an essential component of medical education. *Journal of the Academy of Nutrition and Dietetics*, 117(7), 1104–1113.

Herath, C., Zhou, H., Gan, Y., Nakandawire, N., Gong, Y. *et al.* (2017) A comparative study of interprofessional education in global health care: A systematic review. *Medicine (Baltimore)*, 96(38), e7336.

Kangas, S., Rintala, T.-M. and Jaatinen, P. (2018) An integrative systematic review of interprofessional education on diabetes. *Journal of Interprofessional Care*, 32(6), 706–718.

Khalafalla, F.G., Covarrubias, K., Fesperman, M., Eichmann, K., VanGarsse, A. *et al.* (2020) Enhancing nutrition and lifestyle education for healthcare professional students through an interprofessional, team-based training program. *Currents in Pharmacy Teaching and Learning*, 12(12), 1484–1490.

Kinnison, T. and May, S.A. (2013) Veterinary career ambitions correlate with gender and past experience, with current experience influencing curricular perspectives. *Veterinary Record*, 172(12), 313.

Kinnison, T., Lumbis, R., Orpet, H., Welsh, P., Gregory, S. *et al.* (2011) Piloting interprofessional education interventions with veterinary and veterinary nursing students. *Journal of Veterinary Medical Education*, 38(3), 311–318.

Kinnison, T., Guile, D. and May, S.A. (2015a) Errors in veterinary practice: Preliminary lessons for building better veterinary teams. *Veterinary Record*, 177(19), 492.

Kinnison, T., Guile, D. and May, S.A. (2015b) Veterinary team interactions, part one: The practice effect. *Veterinary Record*, 177(16), 419.

Kinnison, T., May, S.A. and Guile, D. (2015c) Veterinary team interactions part two: The personal effect. *Veterinary Record*, 177, 541.

Kinnison, T., Guile, D. and May, S.A. (2016) The case of veterinary interprofessional practice: From one health to a world of its own. *Journal of Interprofessional Education & Practice*, 4, 51–57.

Kinnison, T., Lumbis, R., de Mestre, A.M. and Cardwell, J.M. (2021) Preliminary testing of psychometric properties of the 'Student Perceptions of Veterinary

Interprofessional Education and Work Scale' (SP-VIEWS). *Journal of Interprofessional Care*, 36(3), 449–457.

Klevans, D.R. and Parrett, J.L. (1990) Continuing professional education needs of clinical dietitians in Pennsylvania. *Journal of the American Dietetic Association*, 90(2), 282–286.

Lingard, L., Reznick, R., Espin, S., Regehr, G. and DeVito, I. (2002) Team communications in the operating room: Talk patterns, sites of tension, and implications for novices. *Academic Medicine: Journal of the Association of American Medical Colleges*, 77(3), 232–237.

Lumbis, R., Langridge, A., Serlin, R. and Kinnison, T. (2021) Developing interprofessional education initiatives to aid working and learning between veterinarians and veterinary nurses/vet techs. *Journal of Veterinary Medical Education*, 48(1), 8–13.

O'Shea, M.-C., Reeves, N.E., Bialocerkowski, A. and Cardell, E. (2019) Using simulation-based learning to provide interprofessional education in diabetes to nutrition and dietetics and exercise physiology students through telehealth. *Advances in Simulation*, 4(S1), 1–8.

Pullon, S., McKinlay, E., Beckingsale, L., Perry, M., Darlow, B. *et al.* (2013) Interprofessional education for physiotherapy, medical and dietetics students: a pilot programme. *Journal of Primary Health Care*, 5(1), 52–58.

Rauch, M., Tipold, A., Wissing, S. and Kleinsorgen, C. (2021) Interprofessional survey on communication skills in veterinary and veterinary-related education in Germany. *BMC Medical Education*, 21(1), 1–12.

Reeves, S., Fletcher, S., Barr, H., Birch, I., Boet, S. *et al.* (2016) A BEME systematic review of the effects of interprofessional education: BEME Guide No. 39. *Medical Teacher*, 38(7), 656–668.

Svensberg, K., Kalleberg, B.G., Rosvold, E.O., Mathiesen, L., Wøien, H. *et al.* (2021) Interprofessional education on complex patients in nursing homes: A focus group study. *BMC Medical Education*, 21(1), 1–11.

WHO (2010) Framework for action on interprofessional education & collaborative practice. Available at: https://www.who.int/publications/i/item/framework-for-action-on-interprofessional-education-collaborative-practice (accessed 19 December 2022).

Conclusion

11

Tierney Kinnison

Abstract
In this concluding chapter regarding an interprofessional approach to nutrition, the main messages of the book are summarised. These include the importance of nutrition as a vital sign and the requirement for frequent consultation with caretakers regarding the nutrition of their pets, our patients. In addition, the chapter reminds us of the benefits of a team whereby individuals are empowered to contribute their own knowledge and skills in an environment which promotes trust, respect and appropriate communication in order to present a united front and enable the veterinary healthcare team (VHCT) as a whole to be the primary providers of nutritional advice to society.

The aim of this book was to share evidence-based suggestions to aid interprofessional working regarding nutrition in veterinary practices. As per the definition of evidence-based veterinary medicine – 'evidence-based decisions combine clinical expertise, the most relevant and best available scientific evidence, patient circumstances and owners' values' (RCVS Knowledge, n.d.) – it is important for each reader to use the scientific evidence presented here considering their own contexts.

It is almost certain, however, at least in the UK, that veterinary practices will employ multiple professions and occupations, and for these to also interact with external experts. Therefore, it is vital to reflect upon interprofessional working, in whatever meaning best suits each reader. It is clear from the literature presented in this volume (as well as from common sense) that different groups working together can pool their knowledge, skills, experience and perspectives, thus leading to a better informed and better skilled group. It is also not surprising that joining together such experts, who bring with them individual factors such as past experience and current status (e.g. owner or employee), means that challenges can arise during interprofessional working. While much research on interprofessional working focuses on one-off events such as behaviour in the operating room during surgeries, a focus on continuing nutritional care of patients in veterinary medicine is highly appropriate.

Nutritional assessment is an important, yet often overlooked, aspect of veterinary care and should be completed for every animal at every visit to determine the most appropriate feeding approach. It is recommended that readers re-visit the World Small Animal Veterinary Association (WSAVA) nutritional assessment guidelines and toolkit as a valuable approach to nutritional assessment. As this book has demonstrated, members of all professions and groups are involved in patients' nutritional assessments and can therefore extend their expertise to the group. To avoid the negative consequences of caretakers potentially following widespread myths and misinformation, the veterinary healthcare team (VHCT) should therefore take an active lead in being the primary source of nutritional advice.

This team approach to nutritional care of our patients requires thought and discussions by each team to utilise the lessons from this volume for the optimal practice-based approach. However, effective teams have many things in common, including using hierarchies to enable transfer of information and resources to all members of a team, while flattening and removing hierarchies which may impede communication. Advice and support should always be sought from the individual with the most experience, rather than due to professional belonging. This is very significant, however it must of course take into account the legalities of veterinary practice in the situation in which the team resides. Teams which differ in their temporal and spatial make up will have to work hard to maintain contact and mutual understanding. Formal interprofessional structures such as joint team meetings can foster this understanding. A good team also has trust and respect as key features which enable the different perspectives each group and individual brings to be utilised in the best way. While both trust and respect must be earned by all team members, they allow for professions and occupations to listen to the advice of others. Listening is an important facet of communication and is one feature of a team which helps those in traditionally lower status groups to 'speak up' regarding caregivers and patient care, leading to the reduction in mistakes and errors.

Nutritional conversations with caregivers are not always seen as paramount or included in consultations, however this volume recommends that this changes. Educating and involving clients in nutritional decisions can foster good relationships between caregivers and the practice as well as leading to the optimum nutritional approach for the patient. These can be challenging conversations, including the discussion of controversial issues, and therefore must be handled with care. It is hoped that the practical advice in this book will aid the healthcare team in approaching such conversations. Nutritional conversations are not one-off events in the life of a patient, and instead range from initial assessments and dietary recommendations through to the delivery of prompt and targeted nutrition, accurate monitoring and provision of pet caretaker advice and support. A clear definition of responsibilities in a VHCT, alongside appropriate delegation and utilisation of all members of the team can help to ensure that all aspects of nutritional care are provided.

While this volume tasks practices with encouraging the continuing professional development (CPD) of their teams regarding nutrition and inter-professional working, the education of future veterinarians and veterinary nurses (VNs) regarding such teamworking should start from day one of their studies. Therefore, interprofessional education (IPE) at both the pre-graduation and post-graduation stage is required, and Chapter 10 offers explanation and examples of IPE for practices and educators in veterinary education settings.

The authors hope that the information contained in this book will enable you, the reader, to foster and enhance the great interprofessional interactions that occur in veterinary practices worldwide, thus ensuring that veterinary healthcare teams are successful providers of nutritional care to animals in our society. In addition to these benefits to our patients, their caretakers, our practices and our healthcare teams will also benefit from an interprofessional approach to veterinary nutrition.

Reference

RCVS Knowledge (n.d.). Available at: https://knowledge.rcvs.org.uk/evidence-based-veterinary-medicine/what-is-ebvm/ (accessed 19 December 2022).

Index

Note: Page numbers in **bold** type refer to **figures**; Page numbers in *italic* type refer to *tables*

collective competence 7
communication 9
    interprofessional 71–76
    problems 115
    VHCT and clients 76–89
        controversial topics 84–87
        enhancing 77–78
        feeding nutrition into
            conversations 77–80
        models of 76–77
        nutritional history, components
            of **79**
        nutritional recommendation
            80–84
        nutrition conversations,
            challenges 88–89
confidentiality and trust 123
    see also trust
consequentialism theories 67
consultation efficiency 77
content failures 72
continuing education (CE) regarding
    nutrition 157
continuing professional development (CPD) 5,
    157, 162, 167
conventional and unconventional food 37
coronavirus pandemic 97
CRAAP (currency, relevance, authority,
    accuracy, purpose) test 22, 27–28
crew resource management (CRM) 2
Critical Appraisal Skills Programme
    (CASP) 30
cultural identity 18

decision-making 67, 77, 130, 144–145
deontology 67
diet/dietary
    assessment 44–45
    choice 88–89
    elimination trial 84
    predilections 18
    -related non-communicable diseases 13
dieticians 1
digital communication and telemedicine 140
disease detection 40
dissatisfaction 53, 150

emotional intelligence 96
empowerment 77, 126, 132, 143, 152
enthusiasm and commitment 138
errors 71–73

ethics/ethical
    of care 67
    consumerism 67
    decision-making 67–68
    dilemmas 67
    pet caretakers' decision-making 68
    vegetarianism and veganism 66
European Board of Veterinary Specialisation
    (EBVS) 87, 144
evidence-based information 86
evidence-based pet dietary
    decision-making 22
evidence-based veterinary medicine 67, 165
experience-based hierarchy 51

face-to-face communication 72
feeding, optimal pet nutrition 18–19, 38
financial constraints 132
'5 As' model 135
flavour preferences 18
follow-up 135, 138
    appointment 129
food sensitivities 84

genetics 13
Global nutrition toolkit 41–42
grass sickness 124–125
guinea pig with malocclusion
    communication 130
    professional roles and
        responsibilities 131–132
    reflection and evaluation 132
    scenario 127–130
    trust and value 130–131
gut feelings, pet food selection 18

heavily-processed commercial pet food 142
hidden curriculum 160
hierarchy
    existence 6
    experience-based 51
    nutrition programme 50–52
    structures 115
honesty and integrity 123
"hub and spoke" model 6
human–animal bond (HAB) 13–14, 130
    veterinary health triangle 15, **15**
Human Animal Bond Research Institute 14
human–animal interactions 13–18
    caretakers' lives **17**